ESSENTIALS OF DENTAL CARIES

A DENTAL PRACTITIONER HANDBOOK
SERIES EDITED BY DONALD D. DERRICK, DDS, LDS RCS

ESSENTIALS OF DENTAL CARIES

The Disease and its Management

EDWINA A. M. KIDD
PhD, BDS, FDS RCS(Eng)

Reader in Conservative Dental Surgery,
United Medical and Dental Schools,
University of London

SALLY JOYSTON-BECHAL
PhD, BDSc, MS, FRACDS

Senior Lecturer,
Department of Oral Medicine and Periodontology,
The London Hospital Medical College Dental School,
University of London

WRIGHT
BRISTOL
1987

Published under the Wright imprint by
IOP Publishing Limited, Techno House, Redcliffe Way, Bristol BS1 6NX, England

British Library Cataloguing in Publication Data

Kidd, Edwina A.M.
Essentials of dental caries: the disease and its management
1. Dental caries
I. Title II. Joyston-Bechal, Sally
617.6′7 RK331

ISBN 0 7236 0842 3

Typeset by
Severntype Repro Services Ltd,
Market Street, Wotton-under-Edge, Gloucestershire

Printed in Great Britain by
Henry Ling Ltd, Dorset Press, Dorchester

PREFACE

When this book was commissioned the request was for a cariology text suitable for the undergraduate. Our aim, therefore, was to produce a book which the junior undergraduate might find easy to read and clinically relevant. By bringing basic theoretical concepts to the chairside we hope that the student will understand the rationale behind the clinical techniques.

We have tried to keep the text simple without being simplistic in the hope that the student will be sufficiently stimulated to use this text as a springboard to the necessary further study. Indeed, there are many other more comprehensive texts and this book seeks to complement them but not to rival them. To this end the use of references has been kept to a minimum. Where possible, review articles or chapters in the more comprehensive texts are referred to, but where such reviews do not exist, more extensive reference lists are included.

On occasions we have tried to highlight areas of ignorance, because current ideas and techniques are not sacred but what today's research and experience suggest. Tomorrow, further research and experience may suggest different solutions to the problems. Indeed the problems themselves may change and a textbook like this will require regular updating.

E. A. M. K.
S. J.-B.

ACKNOWLEDGEMENTS

Several friends have offered constructive criticism which has proved valuable. We would like to thank Mrs T. Barker, Mr J. Buchanan, Dr S. Challacombe, Professor B. Clarkson, Professor R. Duckworth, Dr T. Grenby, Mr Simon Joyston-Bechal, Mr J. Page, Dr G. Roberts, Professor A. Rowe, Dr B. Smith and Dr J. Weinman. Mr N. Taylor willingly assisted with many of the illustrations. The manuscript was typed calmly and accurately by Mrs I. Grubb; her assistance was invaluable. Miss E. Valmorbida designed the cover and we are grateful for her help.

CONTENTS

CHAPTER 1

INTRODUCTION

1.1. DEFINITION OF DENTAL CARIES

Dental caries is a disease of the mineralized tissues of the teeth, namely enamel, dentine and cementum, caused by the action of microorganisms on fermentable carbohydrates. It is characterized by demineralization of the mineral portion of these tissues followed by disintegration of their organic material. The disease can result in bacterial invasion and death of the pulp and spread of infection into the periapical tissues, causing pain. However, in its very early stages the disease can be arrested since it is possible for remineralization to occur.

1.2. AETIOLOGY OF DENTAL CARIES

Some *plaque bacteria* are capable of fermenting a suitable dietary *carbohydrate substrate* (such as the sugars sucrose and glucose) to produce acid, causing the plaque pH to fall to below 5 within 1–3 minutes. Repeated falls in pH in *time* may result in the demineralization of a *susceptible site on a tooth surface,* thus initiating the carious process. The interplay of these four causative factors is sometimes represented diagrammatically by a number of overlapping circles (*Fig.* 1.1). Only when all four factors are present will caries occur.

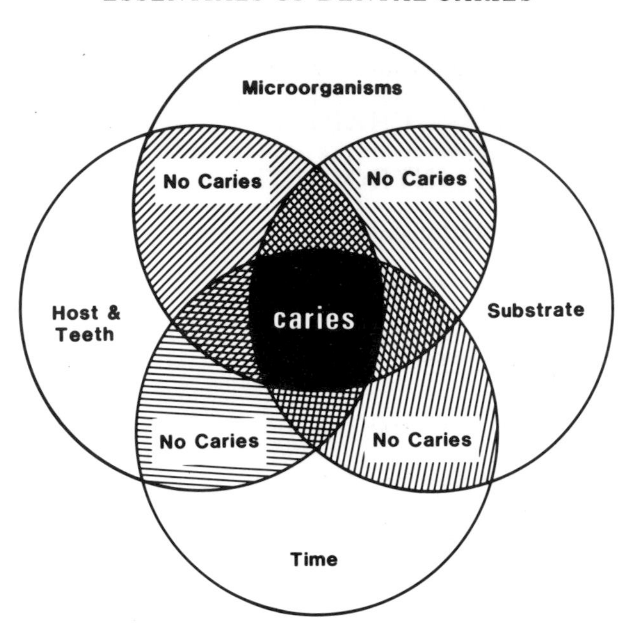

Fig. 1.1. The four circles represent the interplay of the aetiological factors in dental caries. All four factors must be acting simultaneously for caries to occur.

1.2.1. Dental Plaque

Dental plaque is an adherent deposit of bacteria and their products, which forms on all tooth surfaces. It is not an accidental accumulation of bacteria but develops in a sequence of steps.

When a clean enamel surface is exposed to the oral environment it becomes covered with an amorphous organic film called the pellicle. This consists mainly of a glycoprotein precipitated from saliva and begins to form immediately after brushing; it is very tenacious and can attract and help anchor specific kinds of bacteria to the tooth surface.

The organisms which initially colonize the pellicle are predominately coccal in form. A large proportion of these are streptococci. These organisms grow, divide and produce an extracellular gel which is sticky and traps other bacterial forms. Within a few days the plaque becomes thicker and a mixture of different types of microorganisms comprise the bacterial community. Consequently, the flora of the plaque changes from its initial predominantly coccal form to a mixed flora consisting of cocci, rods and filaments.

The Role of Bacteria

In a series of animal experiments in the 1950s, Orland and Keyes and co-workers showed that bacteria were essential for the production of a carious lesion. They fed rodents a highly cariogenic diet and found that they did not develop caries when kept in germ-free conditions. Caries only developed in these animals when bacteria were introduced. In 1960 Keyes infected germ-free animals with known strains of streptococci and found that these organisms were transferred to uninfected litter mates who then became susceptible to caries. He thus demonstrated that dental caries was potentially infectious and transmissible.

In order to establish which organisms were cariogenic, experiments were carried out using rodents with a known flora. (Animals with a known flora are called gnotobiotic.) This work showed that *Streptococcus mutans* and some strains of lactobacilli and actinomycetes were of particular relevance to caries in these animals. Subsequently, such organisms, taken from human lesions, were used to induce caries in previously caries-free monkeys fed a high sugar diet. It was also shown that the organisms, and consequently susceptibility to caries, could be transferred, probably by oral contact, from mother to offspring. However, adult cage-mates were more resistant, perhaps because their oral flora was already established.

Streptococcus mutans and lactobacilli are cariogenic because they are able to produce acid rapidly from fermentable carbohydrates. They thrive under acid conditions and are able to adhere to the tooth surface because of their ability to synthesize sticky extracellular polysaccharides from dietary sugars. These polysaccharides, which are mainly polymers of glucose, give the matrix of dental plaque its gelatinous consistency. Consequently, they help bacteria to stick to each other and to the tooth and, by thickening the layer of plaque, prevent saliva from neutralizing plaque acid.

It has been shown that in mouths of caries-active patients, *S. mutans* and lactobacilli are more numerous than in caries-free individuals. Recent studies in humans have also shown that *S. mutans* can be passed on from mothers to their infants, probably by oral contact. Dental caries should therefore be regarded as an infectious and transmissible disease.

1.2.2. The Role of Dietary Carbohydrate

It is necessary for fermentable carbohydrates and plaque to be present on the tooth surface for a minimum length of time for acid to form and cause demineralization of dental enamel. These carbohydrates provide the plaque bacteria with the substrate for acid production and for the synthesis of extracellular polysaccharides. However, carbohydrates are not all equally cariogenic. While complex carbohydrates such as starch are relatively harmless because they are not completely digested in the mouth, the low molecular weight carbohydrates (sugars) readily diffuse into plaque and are quickly metabolized by the bacteria. Thus, many sugar-containing foods and drinks cause a rapid drop in plaque pH to a level which can cause

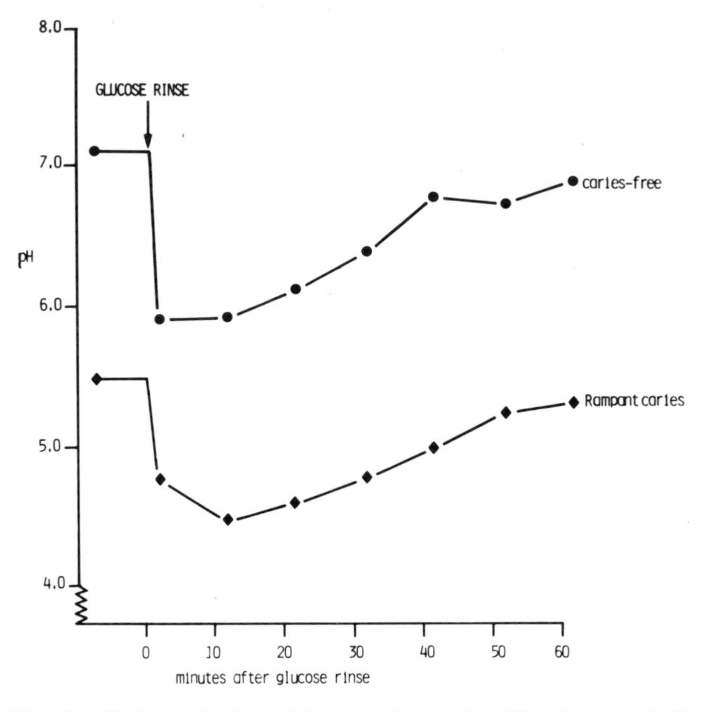

Fig. 1.2. pH changes in plaque following a glucose rinse ('Stephan curve'). The fall in plaque pH is greater in a person with rampant caries than in a caries-free individual.

demineralization of dental enamel. The plaque remains acid for some time, taking 30–60 minutes to return to its normal pH in the region of 7. *Repeated* and *frequent* consumption of sugar will keep plaque pH depressed and cause demineralization of the teeth.

The change in plaque pH may be represented graphically over a period of time following a glucose rinse (*Fig.* 1.2). Such a graph is called a 'Stephan curve' after the person who first described it in 1944. It is interesting that Stephan showed that the fall in plaque pH was greater in a caries-active than in a caries-free individual.

The synthesis of extracellular polysaccharides from sucrose is more rapid than from glucose, fructose and lactose. Consequently, sucrose is the most cariogenic sugar, although the other sugars are also harmful. Since sucrose is also the sugar eaten most commonly, it is the most important cause of dental caries.

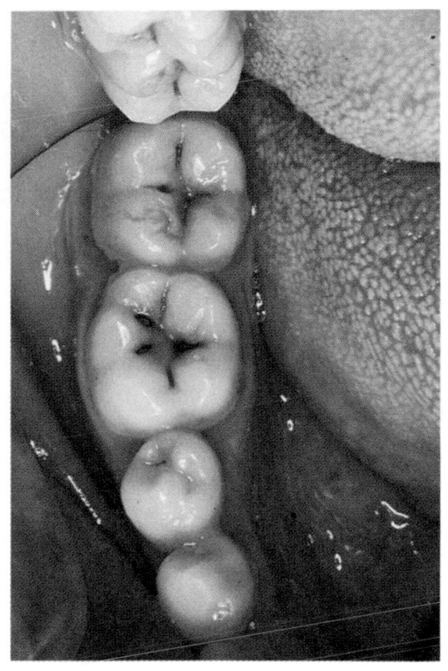

Fig. 1.3. Occlusal caries in molars, showing stained fissures. Cavities were present.

1.2.3. The Susceptibility of the Tooth Surface

Tooth Morphology: Susceptible Sites

Bacterial plaque is a necessary precursor of caries and for this reason sites on the tooth surface which favour plaque retention and stagnation are particularly prone to decay. These sites are:

a. Enamel pits and fissures on occlusal surfaces of molars and premolars (*Fig.* 1.3); buccal pits of molars and palatal pits of maxillary incisors.

b. Approximal enamel smooth surfaces just cervical to the contact point (*Fig.* 1.4).

c. The enamel of the cervical margin of the tooth just coronal to the gingival margin (*Fig.* 1.5 *a–c*).

d. In patients where periodontal disease has resulted in gingival recession, the area of plaque stagnation is on the exposed root surface (*Fig.* 1.6).

e. The margins of restorations, particularly those that are deficient or overhanging.

f. Tooth surfaces adjacent to dentures and bridges which increase the areas where stagnation can occur.

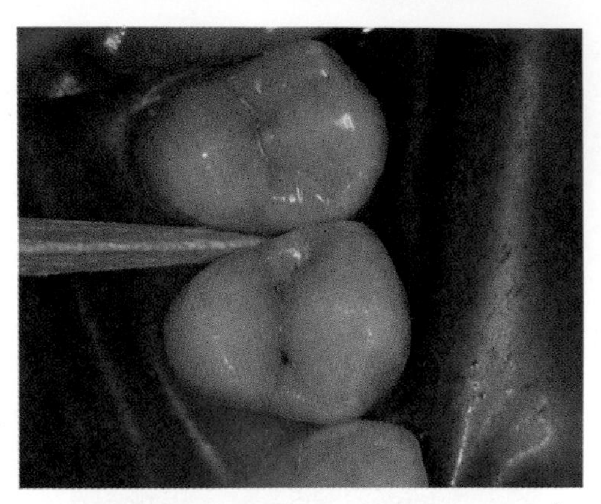

Fig. 1.4. A carious lesion is present on the distal aspect of ⌊4. The lesion is shining up through the marginal ridge which shows a pinkish grey discolouration.

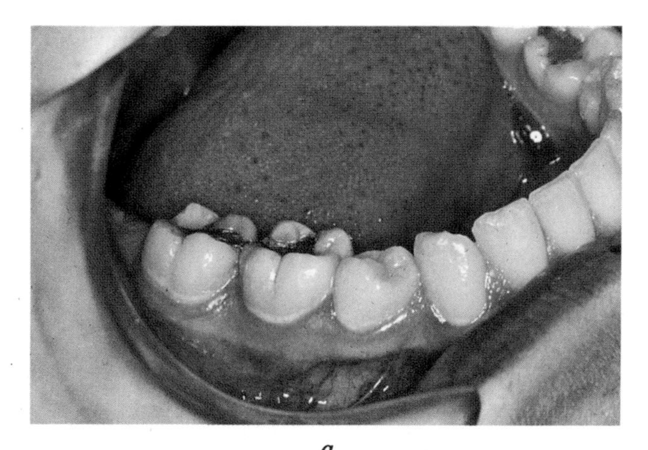

a

Fig. 1.5. *a, b and c.* Caries of the enamel at the cervical margin of $\overline{76|}$. *a.* The white spot lesions covered with plaque. *b.* A red dye has been used to stain the plaque so that the patient can see the plaque clearely. *c.* The patient has now removed the stained plaque with a toothbrush; the white spot lesions are now very obvious. Note they have formed in an area of plaque stagnation.

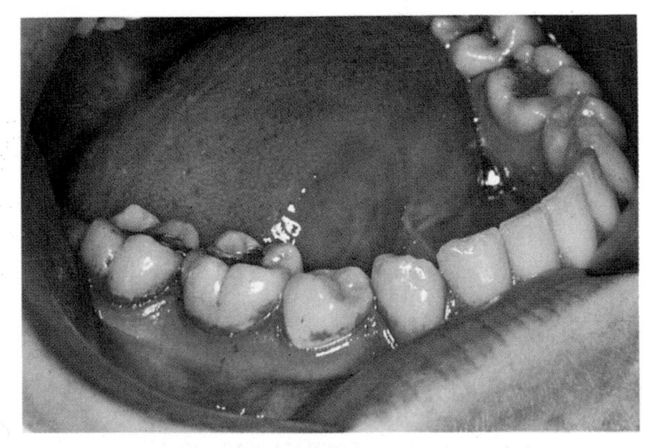

b

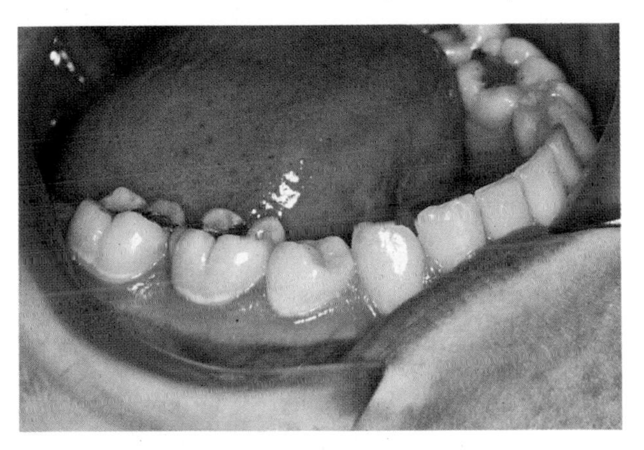

c

The Environment of the Tooth: Saliva, Crevicular Fluid and Fluoride

Under normal conditions, the tooth is continually bathed in saliva. Since the caries susceptibility of the tooth depends to a large extent on its environment, saliva has a considerable part to play (*see* Chapter 5.4). It is capable of remineralizing the early carious lesion because it is supersaturated with calcium and phosphate ions. This remineralizing capacity of saliva is enhanced when the fluoride ion is present. Saliva also influences the pH of plaque as well as the composition of plaque microorganisms. Consequently when salivary flow is greatly diminished or absent, caries may be uncontrolled.

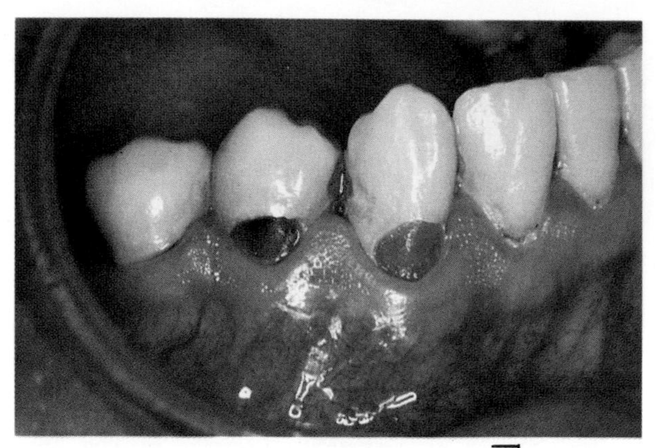

Fig. 1.6. Caries on the exposed root surface buccal to 43⌉.

At the gingival margin the tooth may be washed by crevicular fluid although in the absence of gingival inflammation the volume of fluid is negligible. Crevicular fluid has been shown to contain antibodies, derived from serum, specific to *S. mutans*. The role of these antibodies is currently under investigation but their precise function is yet to be established.

The presence of optimum concentrations of fluoride in the dental tissues and their environment exerts an anticaries effect in several ways (*see* Chapter 7.4). The concentration of fluoride incorporated into the enamel during the process of tooth formation depends on its availability, in the drinking water or in fluoride supplements, for ingestion. Enamel with a higher fluoride content may not in itself be more resistant to acid attack. However, the release of fluoride in the immediate environment during enamel dissolution influences the processes of re- and demineralization, favouring remineralization. In addition, fluoride affects the metabolism of plaque bacteria in relation to acid production.

1.2.4. Time

The ability of saliva to redeposit mineral in the developing carious lesion means that the carious process consists of alternating periods of destruction and repair. Thus, when saliva is present, caries does not destroy the tooth in days or weeks but rather in months or years. Consequently there is a good deal of scope to arrest the disease.

1.3. CLASSIFICATION OF DENTAL CARIES

Caries can be classified according to the anatomical site of the lesion. Thus the lesion may commence in *pits and fissures* or on *smooth surfaces.* Smooth surface lesions may start on enamel or on the exposed root cementum and dentine (*root caries*). Alternatively, caries may develop at the margin of a restoration. This is called *recurrent* or *secondary caries*.

Dental caries may also be classified according to the severity or rapidity of the attack. Different teeth and surfaces are involved depending on the severity of the carious challenge. Thus with a mild challenge only the most vulnerable teeth and surfaces are attacked, such as the occlusal surfaces of permanent molars. A moderate challenge may involve occlusal and approximal surfaces of posterior teeth whereas with a severe challenge anterior teeth, which normally remain caries-free, also become carious. This introduces the concept of *individual variation* of teeth. In addition patients vary in their susceptibility to the disease and in managing dental caries, therefore, it is essential to tailor the treatment to the needs of the individual patient.

Rampant caries is the name given to a sudden rapid destruction of many teeth, frequently involving surfaces of teeth that are ordinarily caries-free. This condition is most commonly observed in the primary dentition of infants who continually suck a dummy or comforter containing, or dipped into, a sugar solution (*Fig.* 1.7). Rampant caries may also be seen in the

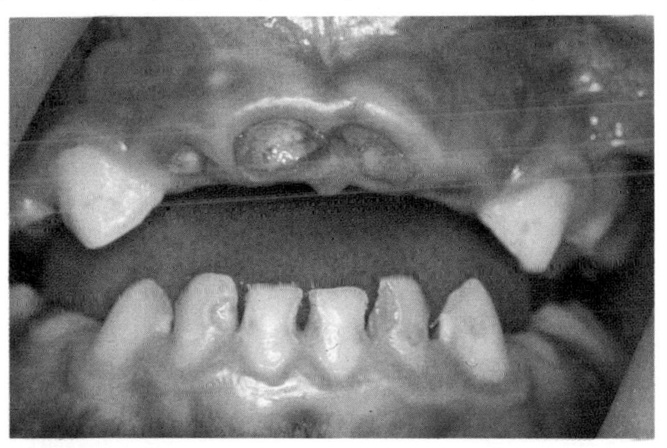

Fig. 1.7. Rampant caries of deciduous teeth. This child continually sucked a dummy filled with rose hip syrup.

permanent dentition of teenagers and is usually due to taking frequent cariogenic snacks and sweet drinks between meals (*Fig.* 1.8). It is also seen in mouths where there is a sudden marked reduction in salivary flow (xerostomia) (*Fig.* 1.9). Radiation in the region of the salivary glands, used in the treatment of a malignant tumour, is the most common cause of an acute xerostomia (*see* Chapter 5.2.2).

In distinct contrast to rampant caries is *arrested caries*. This term describes a carious lesion which does not progress. It is seen when the oral

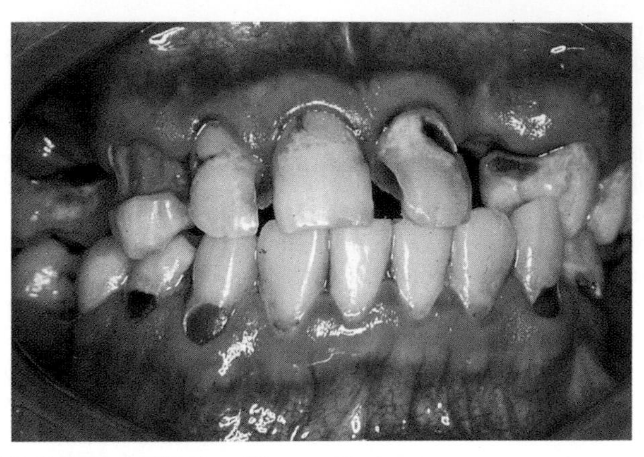

Fig. 1.8. Rampant caries in a 19-year old man.

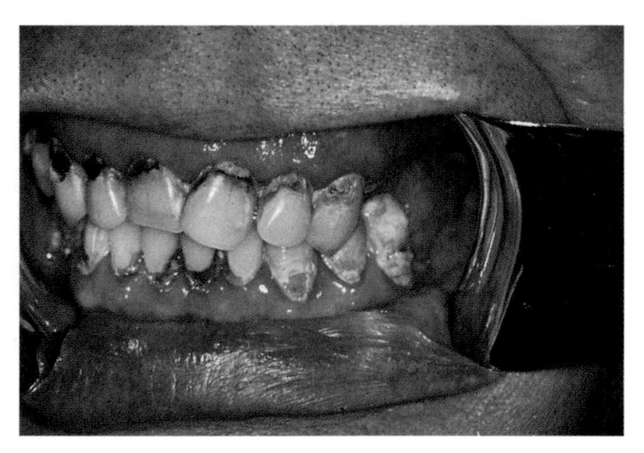

Fig. 1.9. Radiation caries. This patient had been irradiated in the region of the salivary glands for the treatment of a malignant tumour. (By courtesy of Mr F Coffin.)

environment has changed from conditions predisposing to caries to conditions that tend to arrest the lesion. *Fig.* 1.10 shows an arrested lesion on the mesial aspect of a lower second molar. The lesion probably stopped progressing after extraction of the first molar. The environment changed and the surface became more cleansable and accessible to saliva. *Fig.* 1.11 shows a much more advanced carious lesion which has also arrested.

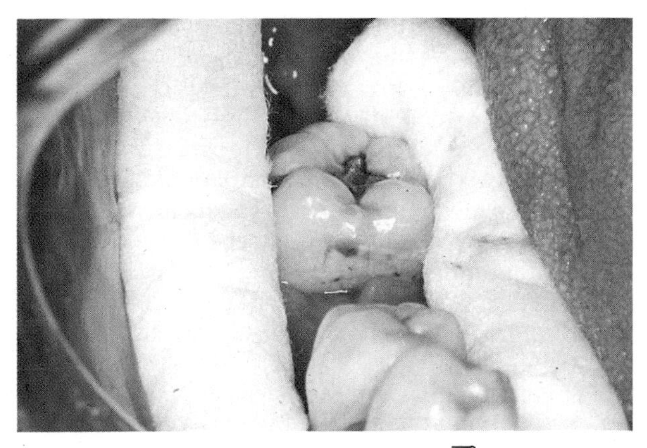

Fig. 1.10. Arrested caries on the mesial aspect of 7⏌. This lesion probably stopped progressing after extraction of 6⏌.

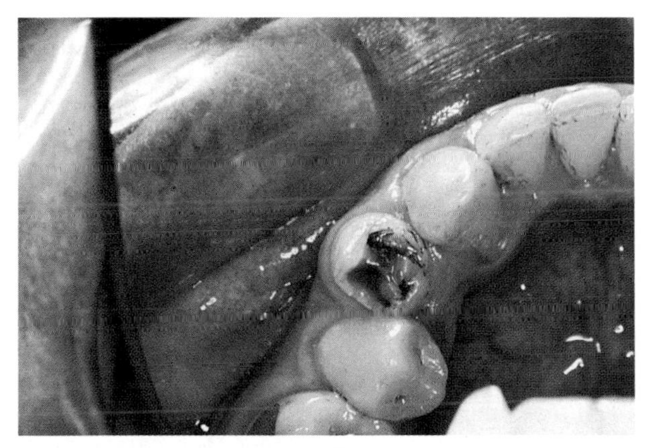

Fig. 1.11. An arrested carious lesion in ⌈4. This lesion was well into dentine, but the tissue was hard and shiny. The tooth had been in this state for at least 10 years.

1.4. EPIDEMIOLOGY OF DENTAL CARIES

Epidemiology is the study of health and disease states in populations rather than individuals. The epidemiologist defines the frequency and severity of health problems in relation to such factors as age, sex, geography, race, economic status, nutrition and diet. It is a bird's-eye view of a problem which attempts to delineate its magnitude, study its cause and assess the efficacy of preventive and management strategies.

1.4.1. Measuring Caries Activity

When studying any disease the epidemiologist is interested in both its *prevalence* and its *incidence.* Prevalence is the proportion of a population affected by a disease or condition at a particular time. Incidence is a measurement of the rate at which a disease progresses. In order to measure incidence, therefore, two examinations are required: one at the beginning and one at the end of a given time period. The incidence of the condition is then the increase or decrease in the number of new cases occurring in a population within that time period.

Before incidence and prevalence can be recorded, a quantitative measurement is required that will reflect accurately the extent of the disease in a population.

In the case of dental caries, the measurements of disease that are used are:

a. the number of decayed teeth with untreated carious lesions (D);
b. the number of teeth which have been extracted and are therefore missing (M);
c. the number of filled teeth (F).

This measurement is known as the DMF index and is an arithmetic index of the cumulative caries attack in a population. DMF(T) is used to denote decayed, missing and filled teeth; DMF(S) denotes decayed, missing and filled surfaces in permanent teeth and therefore takes into account the number of surfaces attacked on each tooth. The similar indices for the primary dentition are def(t) and def(s) where e denotes extracted teeth (to differentiate from loss due to natural exfoliation) and f denotes filled teeth or surfaces.

1.4.2. Practical Problems in DMF and def Indices

There are some potential problems in the use of these indices. In young children, missing deciduous teeth may have been lost due to natural exfoliation and these must be differentiated from those lost due to caries. Permanent teeth are lost for reasons other then caries, such as trauma, extraction for orthodontic purposes and periodontal disease or to facilitate the construction of dentures. Third permanent molars are often removed because there is insufficient room for them in the arch. For this reason, missing teeth may be omitted from the indices and only decayed and filled surfaces included.

The epidemiologist takes enormous trouble to achieve standardization of examination and recording techniques. He will practise and check his diagnoses during a clinical trial to try to ensure reproducibility. Despite this, even the trained and experienced worker will not be completely consistent with himself on the same day, let alone consistent with others in studies spanning years!

In many populations there is a large filled component to the indices and the dentists who have done the fillings are not standardized in their diagnosis of disease. Dentists do not practise and check their diagnostic reproducibility in the same way as epidemiologists. In addition, there is likely to be variation between dentists in their recording of disease. Despite all these problems these indices have been and are of great value in assessing both the prevalence and incidence of dental caries and the effect of various preventive measures.

1.4.3. Caries Prevalence in Modern Man

Dental caries is ubiquitous in modern man living in a highly industrialized society, but caries experience varies greatly between countries and within countries.

Caries prevalence is at present generally lowest for Asian and African countries and highest for the Americas, Europe and Australasia.

1.4.4. Recent Changes in Caries Prevalence

Caries prevalence is increasing rapidly in children in many developing countries. However, in the past 15 years, surveys among schoolchildren in many developed countries have shown a fall in caries prevalence by up to 50 per cent. The studies indicate that there are now more caries-free individuals, fewer decayed surfaces (especially smooth surfaces) and fewer filled teeth.

The reasons for this decline in caries prevalence in developed countries are not fully understood. The following factors may be important:

a. The increased exposure to fluoride in water, in toothpaste and in topical applications in the dental surgery may be of particular importance. The fluoride ion is thought to reduce the incidence of caries in several different ways (*see* Chapter 7.4).

b. A changing pattern of sugar consumption may also be relevant. Since dental caries is a sugar dependent disease, a decrease in frequency and amount of sugar consumed would be expected to affect the prevalence of the disease. Similarly, the increased use of sugar substitutes may be important. These substances impart sweetness but cannot be fermented to acid by bacteria.

c. An improved level of oral health care might influence the disease. Such factors as regular visits to the dentist, improved oral hygiene and increased awareness of the relevance of diet could all be important.

d. A decrease in virulence of the causative organisms may also be relevant. Indeed, this could be of paramount importance because virulence might increase again and thus the prevalence of the disease might increase. It is also possible that the increased use of antibiotics may have affected the causative organisms.

Finding the reasons for any improvement is of more then just academic interest. Until the profession knows why this change has occurred, it will be difficult to predict future patterns. Will the caries rate continue to decrease, stay static or increase again? If the profession has done something right it needs to be indentified and continued! In addition, a knowledge of future patterns of disease has important implications for the planning of dental services for patients.

1.5. DENTAL CARIES IS A PREVENTABLE DISEASE

There is much that can be done to prevent dental caries. Appreciation of the causes of the disease is essential to understanding how it can be prevented. It is also important to regard caries as an alternating process of destruction and repair (*Fig.* 1.12). When the destructive forces outweigh the reparative

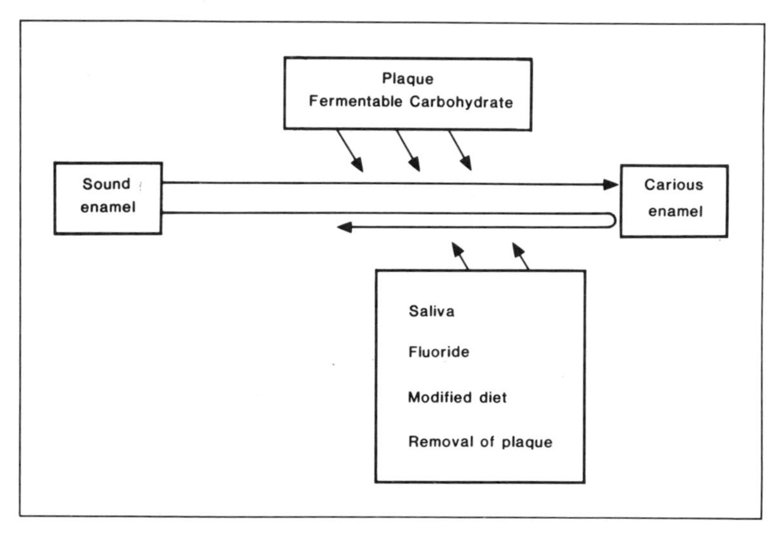

Fig. 1.12. A diagrammatic representation of caries as an alternating process of destruction and repair. Sound enamel will become carious in time if plaque bacteria are given the substrate they need to produce acid. However, saliva is an excellent remineralizing fluid and the arrow can be turned around towards sound enamel again by the use of fluoride, by modifying diet and by attempting to remove plaque.

powers of the saliva the disease will progress (Chapter 5). Conversely, if the reparative forces outweigh the destructive forces, the disease will arrest or even reverse, provided it is caught in its early stages. Consequently, early diagnosis of the disease is of paramount importance (Chapter 4) because if destruction is allowed to proceed too far, only operative intervention can replace the tissue (Chapter 10). Unfortunately, fillings do not prevent caries and new lesions can develop adjacent to restorations (Chapter 11). If fillings are to last, preventive dentistry must go hand in hand with operative dentistry.

The basis of caries prevention is modification of one or more of the three main factors involved in the aetiology of the disease: dental plaque, a suitable carbohydrate substrate and the susceptibility of the host (*see Fig.* 1.1). Since the carious process usually takes months or years to destroy the tooth, time is on the patient's side. Theoretically the three ways of preventing caries are:

a. Eliminate the carbohydrate substrate. Fortunately, complete elimination of refined carbohydrate from the diet is not necessary for the prevention of caries but relatively simple measures, such as reducing the frequency of consumption of sugar and confining it to mealtimes, are usually sufficient (Chapter 6). This is the most effective way of preventing caries.

b. Increase the resistance of the host. Enamel and exposed dentine can be made more resistant to dental caries by appropriate exposure to fluoride (Chapter 7). Deep pits and fissures can be made less susceptible by obliterating or 'sealing' them with a resin (Chapter 8). Since specific microorganisms appear to be involved in the carious process it is possible that in future years individuals may be immunized against this particular infection (Chapter 9). Indeed, a great deal of research effort is currently directed towards this end. However, clinical trials in human subjects have yet to be carried out and even if they were to be successful the advent of immunization on a large scale would still be several years away.

c. Eliminate bacterial plaque. Theoretically a plaque-free tooth surface will not decay but regular complete elimination of plaque is impracticable. Fortunately, not all the bacteria in plaque are capable of fermenting sugar so it may be possible to prevent caries by reducing the numbers of cariogenic bacteria (Chapter 9).

It is salutary to note that each of these preventive measures requires the patient's cooperation. Ultimately it is the patient who will prevent disease, not the dentist. The principle role of the profession, therefore, may be to provide patients with knowledge so that they understand their essential role in disease control. In addition, patients need to be persuaded to accept responsibility for their own mouths (Chapter 12).

However, before discussing the management of dental caries, the disease itself must be understood. The following two chapters describe caries in enamel and dentine and are part of the scientific basis on which management strategies rest.

CHAPTER 2

CARIES IN ENAMEL[1]

2.1. MACROSCOPIC FEATURES OF THE 'EARLY' ENAMEL LESION

The earliest macroscopic evidence of enamel caries is known as the 'white spot lesion'. It is best seen on dried, extracted teeth where the lesion appears as a small, opaque, white area just cervical to the contact point. The colour of the lesion distinguishes it from the adjacent sound enamel. At this stage it cannot be detected with a probe because the enamel overlying the white spot is hard and shiny. Sometimes this lesion may appear brown in colour due to exogenous material absorbed into its porosities (*Fig.* 2.1).

Both white and brown spot lesions may have been present in the mouth for some years, as it is not inevitable for a carious lesion to progress. *Figs.* 1.10 and 2.2 are both examples of lesions which have probably been present for many years and are now static, or 'arrested'. In *Fig.* 1.10 the lesion on the approximal aspect of the second lower molar probably arrested after the first molar was extracted. The area became more accessible to saliva and the toothbrush so that conditions did not favour continued disease. In *Fig.* 2.2 buccal lesions are present. It is likely that these lesions developed soon after the eruption of the tooth in an area of plaque stagnation near the gingival margin. However, the gingival tissues are now positioned closer to the enamel–dentine junction following passive eruption of the tooth. The lesions are now easily accessible for cleaning and are not progressing.

The fact that in its early stages the carious lesion can be arrested implies that efforts should be directed towards early diagnosis and prevention of further disease. However, if the early enamel lesion progresses, the intact surface breaks down (cavitation) and a hole is formed (a cavity).

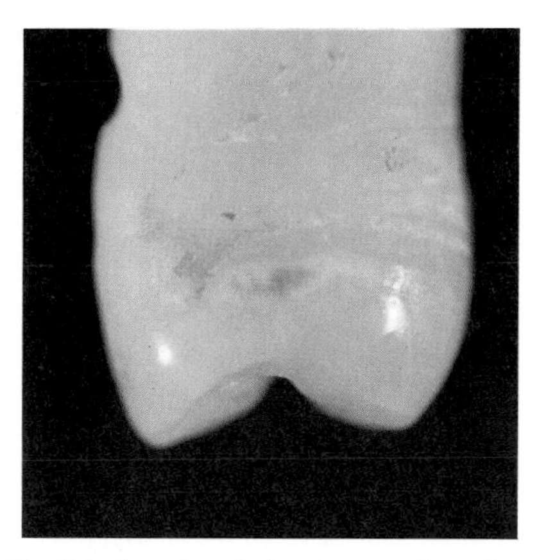

Fig. 2.1. A carious lesion in enamel on the approximal surface of an upper premolar. This lesion is not detectable with a probe but its colour (white and brown) distinguishes it from the adjacent sound enamel.

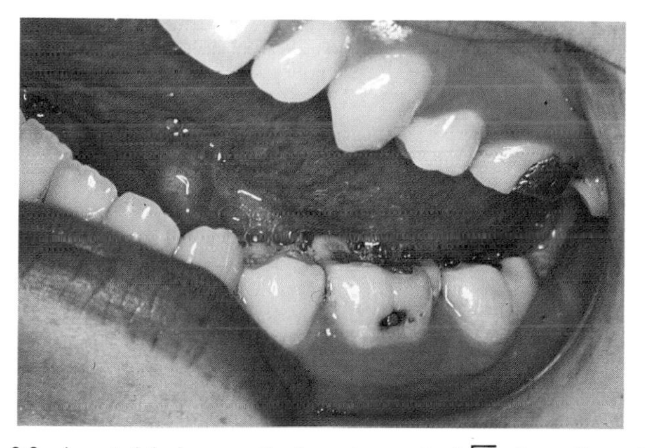

Fig. 2.2. Arrested lesions on the buccal aspect of ⌈6. A small amalgam restoration is also present.

2.2. MICROSCOPIC FEATURES OF THE 'EARLY' ENAMEL LESION

Histological studies have played an important part in the realization that dental caries is not simply a process of progressive demineralization but an alternating process of destruction and repair. In addition, histological studies have shown the pattern of spread of caries. Since management strategies are based on these concepts, a detailed description of the histological features of the lesion will follow.

Four principal methods of examination have been used: light microscopy, microradiography, transmission electron microscopy and scanning electron microscopy.

2.2.1. Light Microscopy—Smooth Surface Lesions

To examine carious enamel in the light microscope, ground sections are required. These sections are cut with a diamond wheel and are then made thinner by grinding on a flat glass surface in a slurry of alumina powder and water. Once a section has been reduced to 100 μm (1 000 μm = 1mm) it is ready to be examined by transmitted light.

Although plain transmitted light can be used, polarized light is often preferred because the lesion is seen particularly clearly. In addition, the polarizing microscope can be used quantitatively to deduce the degree of demineralization of carious enamel.

On a smooth surface, such as the approximal or buccal, the lesion is usually cone shaped, the apex of the cone pointing towards the enamel–dentine junction (*Fig.* 2.3*a*).

The small lesion has been divided into zones[1] based upon its histological appearance when longitudinal ground sections are examined with the light microscope. Four zones may be distinguished. There is a *translucent zone* at the inner advancing front of the lesion, while a *dark zone* may be found just superficial to this. The *body of the lesion* is the third zone lying between the dark zone and the apparently undamaged surface enamel. This zone makes up the major part of the lesion and shows the most marked demineralization. The relatively unaffected *surface zone* superficial to the lesion is the fourth zone. The appearance of each of these four zones of enamel caries in polarized light will now be described.

Zone 1: The Translucent Zone

The translucent zone of enamel caries is not seen in all lesions but when it is present it lies at the advancing front of the lesion and is the first recognizable alteration from normal. This zone is only seen when a longitudinal ground section is examined in a clearing agent, such as quinoline, having the same refractive index (1·62) as that of enamel. The translucent zone appears structureless, the translucency being demarcated from normal enamel on its deep aspect and the dark zone on its superficial aspect (*Fig.* 2.3*b*).

The translucent zone is a more porous region than sound enamel, the pores having been created by the demineralization process. Sound enamel has a pore volume of about 0·1 per cent. The translucent zone, however, has a pore volume of approximately 1 per cent. The pores are probably located at junctional sites such as prism borders, cross striations and along striae of

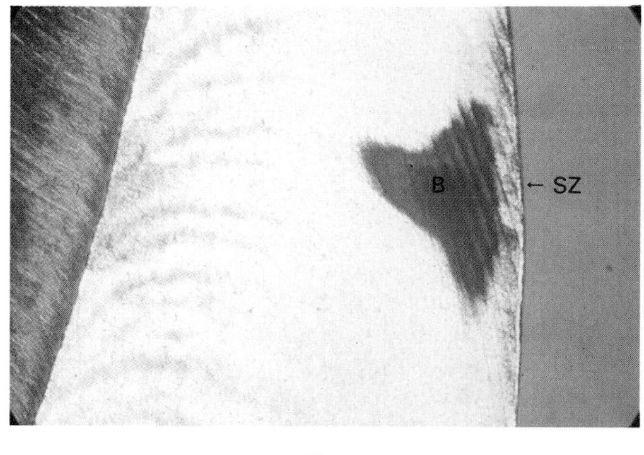

a

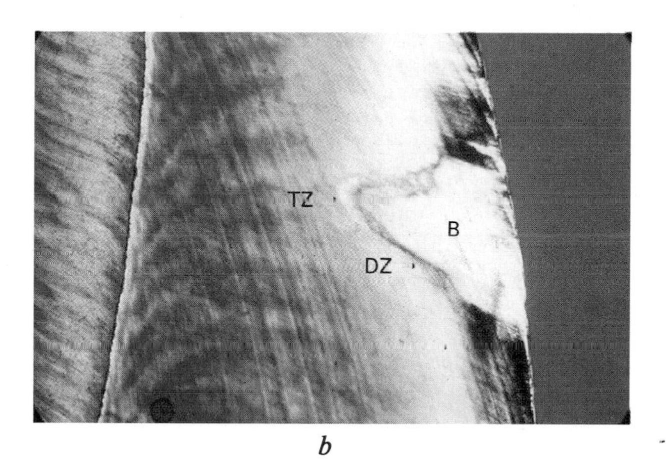

b

Fig. 2.3. *a.* Longitudinal ground section through a small lesion of enamel caries on a smooth surface examined in water with polarized light. The lesion is cone shaped. The body of the lesion (B) appears dark beneath a relatively intact surface zone (SZ). (Magnification × 135.) *b.* The same section as in *a* now examined in quinoline with the polarizing microscope. A translucent zone (TZ) is present at the advancing front of the lesion and a dark zone (DZ) can be seen superficial to this. The body (B) of the lesion appears translucent with well marked striae of Retzius. (Magnification × 135.)

Retzius. Once these areas fill with quinoline structural markings are lost, due to the penetration of a medium having an identical refractive index to that of enamel apatite. This is why the translucent zone looks translucent.

Zone 2: The Dark Zone

If a translucent zone is present at the advancing front of a lesion when examined in quinoline, the dark zone is the second zone of alteration from normal enamel and lies just superficial to the translucent zone. The zone appears dark when the ground section is placed in quinoline (*Fig.* 2.3*b*).

The dark zone is more porous than the translucent zone, having a pore volume of 2–4 per cent. The evidence explaining why the dark zone appears dark is intriguing. It would seem that in this zone the pores are of varying sizes, large and small. Quinoline is a large molecule and cannot enter the small pores which remain filled with air, giving a dark appearance.

There are two theoretical ways in which these small pores may have formed. They may have been created by demineralization, that is by an opening up of sites not previously attacked. Alternatively, the small pores could represent areas of healing where mineral has been redeposited. There is now considerable evidence to support the view that the dark zone can represent an area of remineralization. If arrested lesions, which have been present clinically for many years, are examined histologically, they show wide, well developed dark zones at the front of the lesion, within the body of the lesion and at the surface of the lesion (*Fig.* 2.4).

In addition, attempts have been made to remineralize enamel lesions in the laboratory using human saliva and calcifying fluids prepared from synthetic hydroxyapatite with added fluoride. After exposure there were changes in the histological appearances of the lesions including significant broadening of the dark zones.

Zone 3: The Body of the Lesion

The body of the lesion comprises the largest proportion of carious enamel in the small lesion. It lies superficial to the dark zone and deep to the relatively unaffected surface layer of the lesion. When a longitudinal ground section is examined in quinoline in polarized light, the area appears translucent and the striae of Retzius may be well marked (*Fig.* 2.3*b*).

The body of the lesion is seen particularly clearly if the ground section is examined in water (*Fig.* 2.3*a*). The water molecules enter the pores in the tissue and since the refractive index of water is different to that of enamel, the area appears dark. The pore volume of this region is 5 per cent at its periphery, increasing to 25 per cent or more in the centre.

Zone 4: The Surface Zone

One of the important characteristics of enamel caries is that the small lesion remains covered by a surface layer which appears relatively unaffected by the attack. The zone is most clearly seen in polarized light when the section is in water where it appears as a relatively unaffected area superficial to the body of the lesion (*Fig.* 2.3*a*). The zone has a pore volume of

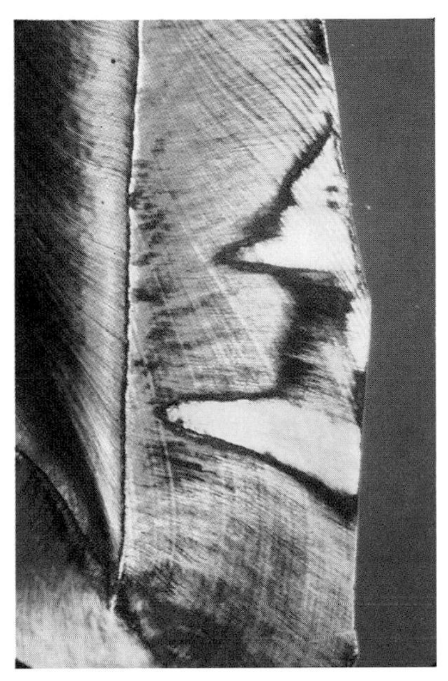

Fig. 2.4. Longitudinal ground section of an arrested caries lesion in a tooth extracted from a patient of 65 years. The section is examined in quinoline with polarized light and shows wide, well developed dark zones at the advancing front of the lesion, within the body of the lesion and at the surface of the lesion. (Magnification × 135.)

approximately 1 per cent, but if the lesion progresses the surface layer is eventually destroyed and a cavity forms.

The subsurface demineralization that characterizes the 'early' enamel lesion has intrigued research workers for many years.[2] Some have suggested that the formation of this relatively unaffected surface layer is associated with the special properties of surface enamel which shows a high degree of mineralization, a higher fluoride content and possibly a greater amount of insoluble protein than subsurface enamel. However, a surface zone can also be produced when the original enamel surface has been ground away. Consequently the existence of surface enamel with 'special' characteristics cannot be entirely responsible.

The surface zone has also been attributed to the presence of a layer of plaque over the lesion. It is suggested that the plaque acts as a diffusion barrier, trapping calcium, phosphate and fluoride ions released by subsurface dissolution or from saturated solution in plaque. These ions may then reprecipitate into the surface enamel. This suggestion implies that the surface zone of enamel caries may, in part, be a manifestation of remineralization.

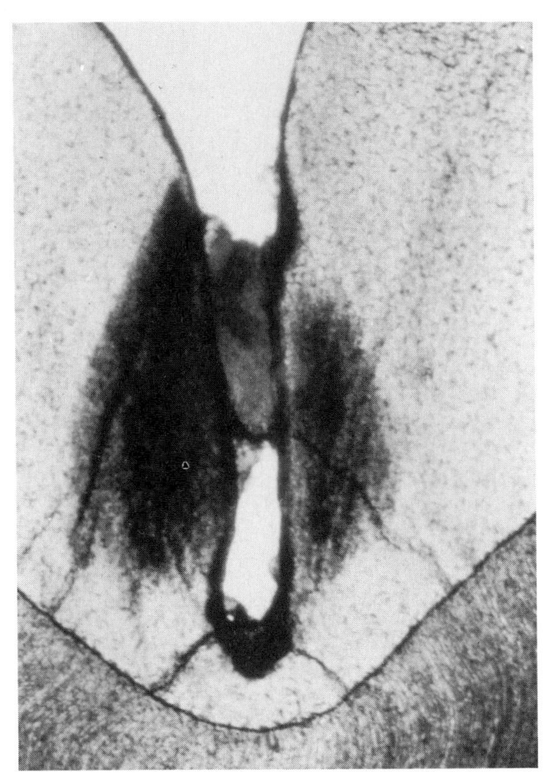

Fig. 2.5. A longitudinal ground section through an occlusal fissure showing a small carious lesion. The section is in water and viewed in transmitted light. The lesion forms on the fissure walls giving the appearance of two smooth surface lesions. (Magnification × 90.)

2.2.2. Light Microscopy—Fissure Caries

Occlusal fissures and buccal pits are obvious stagnation areas where plaque can form and mature, anatomically protected from the toothbrush filament by the minute dimensions of the fissure.

The histological features of fissures caries are similar to those already described for smooth surfaces. The lesion forms around the fissure walls and gives the appearance of two small, smooth surface lesions (*Fig.* 2.5). Eventually the lesions increase in size, coalescing at the base of the fissure. The enamel lesion broadens as it approaches the underlying dentine, guided by prism direction. With lateral spread at the enamel–dentine junction, the area of involved dentine is larger than with smooth surface lesions.

Clinically this is of considerable importance and explains the wide undermining of sound enamel in occlusal caries.

2.2.3. The 'Early' Enamel Lesion in Deciduous Teeth

The histological features of enamel caries in deciduous teeth are similar to those already described in permanent enamel. However, the enamel in deciduous teeth is much thinner than in permanent teeth and the pulps are relatively large. For this reason early diagnosis of caries in primary enamel is of particular importance.

2.2.4. Microradiography

In the laboratory it is possible to take a radiograph of a ground section. This is called a microradiograph and it may be examined in the light microscope.

The technique will demonstrate demineralization in excess of 5 per cent as a radiolucent area (*Fig.* 2.6) which corresponds almost exactly with the body of the lesion as seen in polarized light when the section is in water. A well mineralized radio-opaque surface layer is obvious.

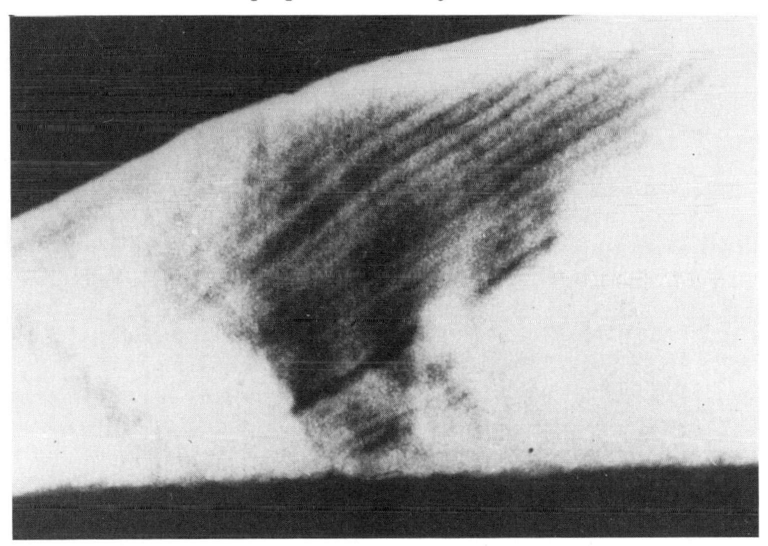

Fig. 2.6. A microradiograph of a ground section showing a carious lesion in the enamel. The body of the lesion shows marked radiolucency and the striae of Retzius can be clearly seen. Superficially the surface of the enamel appears well mineralized. (Magnification × 90.)

2.2.5. Electron Microscopy

The first evidence of a change from sound enamel that can be recognized with the *transmission electron microscope* appears to coincide with the

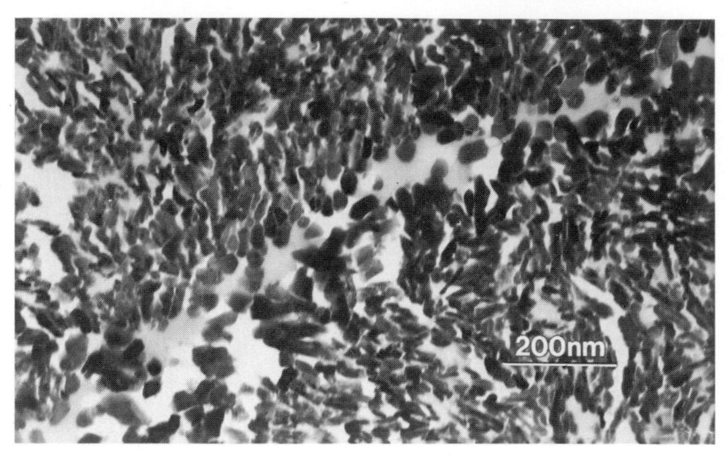

Fig. 2.7. Electron micrograph showing parts of two transversely sectioned prisms from carious enamel. A double row of enlarged, polyhedral crystals is present at the prism junction lining a channel which is largely artefact, but which does contain Araldite embedding medium. The majority of the crystals are irregular flattened hexagons with central deficiencies. (By courtesy of Professor N. W. Johnson.)

body of the lesion as seen in the light microscope. Demineralization of enamel is diffuse affecting both intra- and inter-prismatic enamel. Prism junctions would appear to be sites of preferential dissolution, narrow channels occurring between prisms. In these areas crystallites larger than those in sound enamel may be seen, and these probably represent areas of recrystallization (*Fig.* 2.7). Carious destruction of individual crystals results in loss of crystal centres and in surface damage.

Recently a technique has been developed[3] in which ground sections of white spot lesions have been examined by polarized light and then sectioned with a scalpel. The fractured edges of these pieces have been examined in the *scanning electron microscope* and the diameter of the crystals in sound enamel and in each of the four zones of enamel caries, as seen in the light microscope, has been measured.

These measurements have shown that crystal diameters for sound enamel range from 30–40 nm (nm = nanometre; 1 000 nanometres = 1 micron; 1000 microns = 1 millimetre, i.e. 1 000 000 nm = 1 mm). In the translucent zone of the enamel lesion crystal diameters were smaller than for sound enamel and varied from 25 to 30 nm. In the dark zone, however, crystal diameters were significantly greater than sound enamel, being 50–100 nm, while in the body of the lesion crystal diameters were found to be much smaller, in the range of 10–30 nm. In the surface zone, crystal

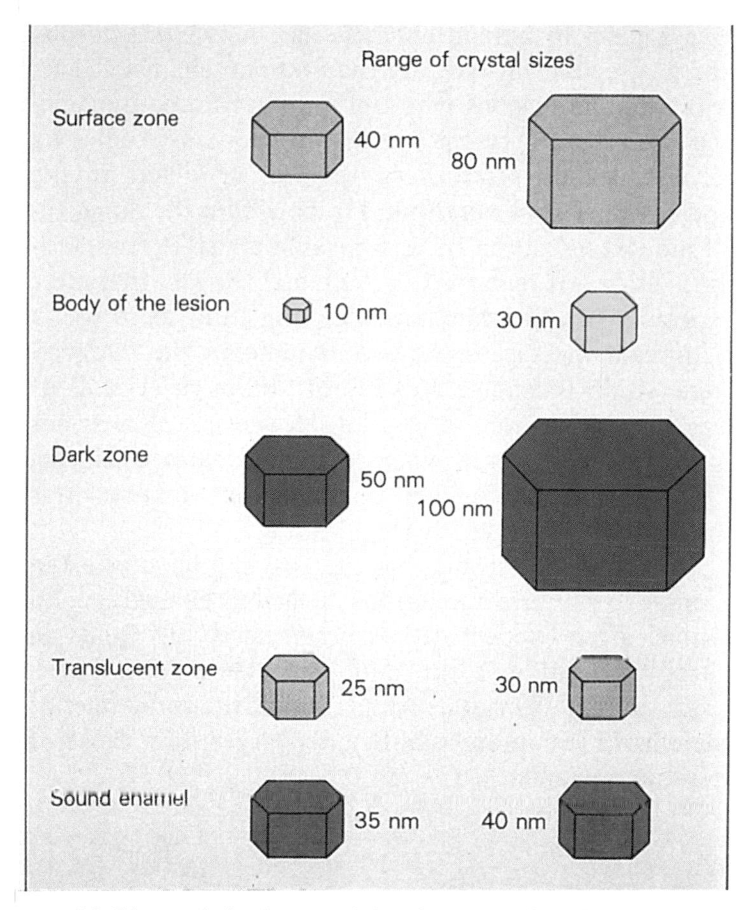

Fig. 2.8. Diagram indicating crystal sizes found in all four of the histological zones of enamel caries. (Reproduced from Silverstone L. M. (1983) *Dent. Update* **10**, 261–273, with permission of publishers and author.)

diameters were once again found to be larger than in sound enamel, being in the range 40–80nm (*Fig.* 2.8).

The fact that the crystal diameters in the dark zone and the surface zone are larger than in sound enamel is important because it is direct evidence that dental caries is not just a process of demineralization but that remineralization can also occur. During the remineralizing process these crystals have grown to be larger than those in unblemished sound enamel.

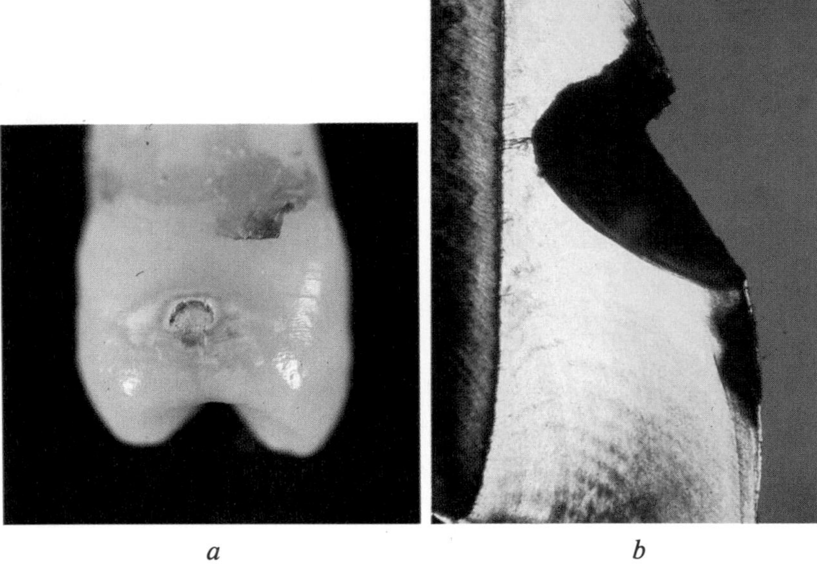

a b

Fig. 2.9. *a.* A cavitated enamel lesion on the approximal surface of a premolar tooth. *b.* A longitudinal ground section through this lesion examined in water with the polarizing microscope.

2.3. REMINERALIZATION

Remineralization may be defined as the deposition of mineral or inorganic substances in an area from which such substances were previously removed. It is very important to realize that dental caries is characterized by alternating periods of destruction and repair. Fortunately, teeth are bathed in saliva which is a remineralizing fluid. Thus clinicians can help patients tip the balance in favour of repair if they are able to detect enamel caries in its earliest form and then institute the relevant preventive measures. Unfortunately, once cavitation occurs, remineralization will not 'fill up the hole'. For this reason the clinician must make every effort to detect the white spot lesion (*see* Chapter 4).

There is now some evidence that remineralized enamel lesions may be more resistant to a further acid attack than sound enamel. Thus a 'healed' white spot lesion may be regarded as scar tissue and should certainly not be attacked with a dental drill. There may be several reasons for its toughness. The fact that it contains crystals that are larger than sound enamel may be relevant as such crystals will take longer to dissolve. In addition, the lesion has a high fluoride content since porous enamel takes up fluoride readily from any fluoride in its environment, such as fluoridated toothpaste or water. Finally, the relatively high protein content of the tissue may also be protective.

2.4. CAVITATION

If, on the other hand, the lesion progresses, the surface zone eventually breaks down and a cavity forms (*Fig.* 2.9*a* and *b*). Plaque now forms within the cavity and may be protected from cleaning aids such as a toothbrush filament or dental floss. For this reason a cavitated lesion is more likely to progress, although it can still arrest and partially remineralize, especially if diet is changed and the cariogenic microorganisms are starved of their substrate or if it is on a surface which is accessible to a toothbrush.

REFERENCES

1. Silverstone L. M. (1973) The structure of carious enamel, including the early lesion. In: Melcher and Zarb (ed.), *Oral Sciences Reviews, No. 4. Dental Enamel.* Copenhagen, Munksgaard, pp. 100–160.
2. Thylstrup A. and Fejerskov O. (1986) *Textbook of Cariology.* Copenhagen, Munksgaard, Chapter 10.
3. Silverstone L. M. (1983) Remineralization and enamel caries: new concepts. *Dent. Update* **10**, 261–273.

CHAPTER 3

CARIES IN DENTINE AND ITS EFFECT ON THE PULP[1]

3.1. SHAPE OF LESIONS: SMOOTH SURFACE AND FISSURE

It has been emphasized in Chapter 2 that enamel carious lesions on smooth surfaces and in fissures differ in shape because of the anatomy of the fissure and the direction of the enamel prisms. The smooth surface lesion is cone shaped, the base of the cone being at the enamel surface. The fissure lesion is also ultimately cone shaped but the base of the cone is at the enamel–dentine junction. This is because the spread of the enamel lesion is guided by prism direction and hence the fissure lesion broadens as it approaches the dentine.

When and if the carious process reaches the enamel–dentine junction, caries spreads laterally along the junction to involve the dentine on a wider front. This results in the undermining of sound enamel by the carious process and the resulting lesion is larger than would be expected from

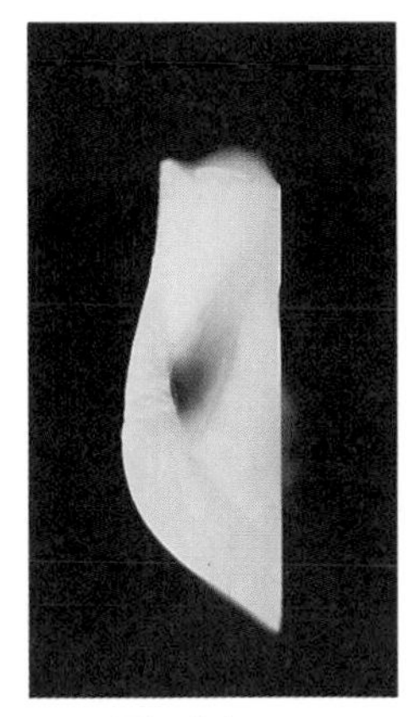

Fig. 3.1.

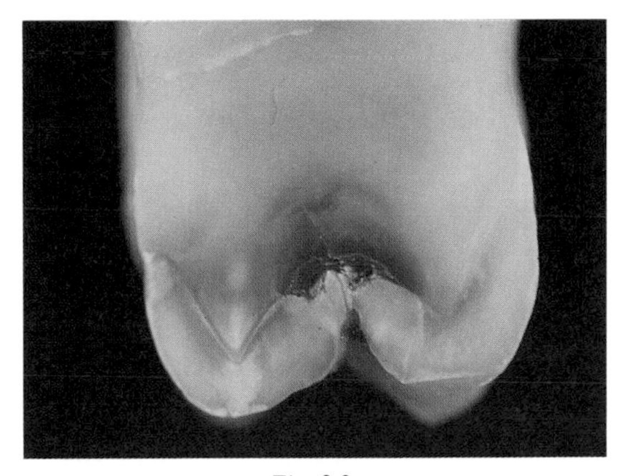

Fig. 3.2

Fig. 3.1. A hemisection of an approximal carious lesion. Note lateral spread of caries along the enamel–dentine junction. In dentine the carious process follows the dentinal tubules.

Fig. 3.2. A hemisection of a carious lesion in a fissure. The enamel lesion has formed bilaterally on the walls of the fissure. Lateral spread along the enamel–dentine junction has resulted in extensive undermining of the enamel. The clinical appearance of this lesion was similar to *Fig.* 1.3.

examination of the enamel alone, particularly in fissure lesions (*Fig.* 3.1 and *Fig.* 3.2).

Undermined enamel tends to be brittle and may eventually fracture under occlusal forces to produce a large cavity. The undermining of sound enamel by the carious process is of particular relevance in cavity preparation because enamel must often be removed to gain access to the carious dentine beneath it. In addition, it is thought to be unwise to leave undermined enamel in areas of occlusal stress because the forces of occlusion may fracture it. For this reason, lateral spread of caries along the enamel–dentine junction is one of the main determinants of cavity size (*see* Chapter 10).

3.2. THE PULP–DENTINE COMPLEX

Dentine is a vital tissue containing the cytoplasmic extensions of the odontoblasts in the dentinal tubules. The odontoblast cell bodies line the pulp chamber and their continued vitality is dependent on the blood supply and lymphatic drainage of the pulp tissue. Thus dentine must be considered together with pulp since the two tissues are so intimately connected. The pulp–dentine complex, like any other vital tissue in the body, is capable of defending itself. The state of the tissue at any time will depend on the state of the balance between the attacking forces and the defence reactions.

3.3. POTENTIAL CAUSES OF PULPAL INJURY

Dental caries is not the only cause of pulpal injury;[2] however, the defence reactions of the tissue are the same irrespective of the stimulus.

The stimuli which may invoke the defence reactions include *bacteria* as in dental caries, and *mechanical* stimuli, such as trauma, tooth fracture, cavity preparation and tooth wear. In addition, *chemical* stimuli are important, for example, acids in foods, toxic dental restorative materials and dehydration of dentine which is particularly likely during cavity preparation. Finally, *thermal* shocks, such as excess heat generated by careless use of rotary instruments during cavity preparation or temperature changes transmitted to dentine through large metal restorations from hot or cold foods can be damaging.

3.4. DEFENCE REACTIONS OF THE PULP–DENTINE COMPLEX

The following defence reactions are of importance:

a. tubular sclerosis within the dentine;
b. reactionary dentine at the interface between dentine and pulp;
c. inflammation of the pulp.

Note that all these defence reactions depend on the presence of a vital pulp.

3.4.1. Tubular Sclerosis

Tubular sclerosis (*Fig.* 3.3) is a process in which mineral is deposited within the lumina of the dentinal tubules and may be thought of as an extension of the normal mechanism of peritubular dentine formation.

The response, which requires the action of vital odontoblasts, is commonly seen at the periphery of carious lesions in dentine. Tubular sclerosis results in the affected area being structurally more homogeneous. For this reason there is less scattering of light as it passes through the tissue and the area of dentine is called a *translucent zone.* The term ‘translucent zone’ should not be confused with the translucent zone of enamel caries. In the enamel lesion the translucent zone represents demineralization whereas in the dentine lesion it represents increased mineral content!

Tubular sclerosis may be protective in that it reduces the permeability of the tissue, thus potentially inhibiting the penetration of acids and bacterial toxins.

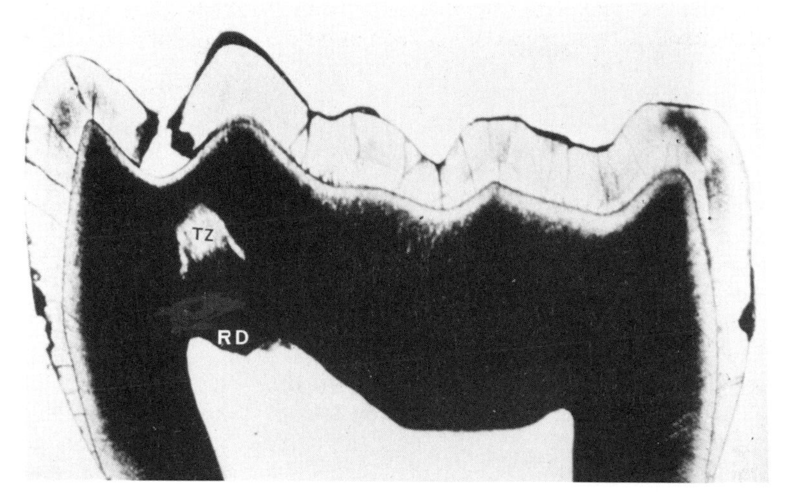

Fig. 3.3. A ground section of a molar crown viewed in transmitted light. A fissure lesion is present. The enamel is cavitated. Tubular sclerosis is seen as a translucent zone in the dentine (TZ). Reactionary dentine (RD) is also present since the pulp horn is partially obliterated. (By courtesy of Professor N. W. Johnson.)

3.4.2. Reactionary Dentine

Reactionary or reparative dentine (*Fig.* 3.4) is a layer of dentine formed at the interface between the dentine and pulp. It is formed in response to a stimulus acting further peripherally and for this reason its distribution is limited to the area beneath the stimulus.

Reactionary dentine should be distinguished from primary dentine which is formed before tooth eruption and secondary dentine which forms throughout life.

Reactionary dentine varies in structure from a well formed tissue with evenly placed tubules indistinguishable from the adjacent primary and secondary dentine, through varying degrees of irregularity in the tubules and degrees of mineralization, to an abnormally formed tissue with few tubules and numerous interglobular areas and even entrapped odontoblasts.

Regular reactionary dentine forms in response to a mild stimulus but with increasing severity of the stimulus there is increasing likelihood of damage to the odontoblasts and dysplasia of the reactionary tissue formed. An overwhelming stimulus can result in death of the odontoblasts and, in this case, no reactionary dentine will be formed. However, sometimes other cells in the pulp differentiate to form an atubular calcified material.

It is thought that the blood supply to the pulp is an important factor determining its ability to produce reactionary dentine. Reactionary dentine

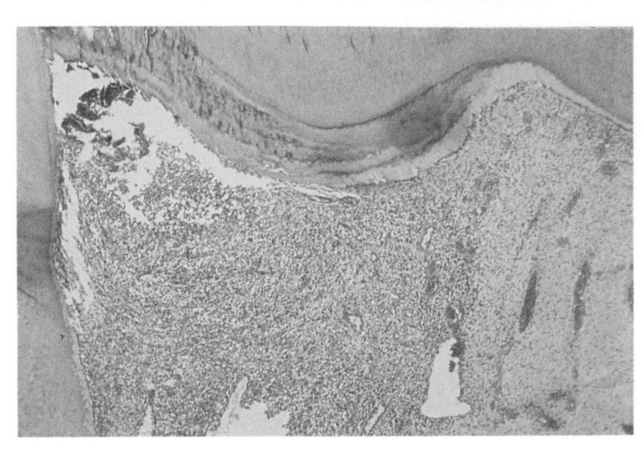

Fig. 3.4. Chronic pulpitis as indicated by the reactionary dentine formation. A predominantly chronic (mononuclear) inflammatory infiltrate is gradually extending across and has largely replaced the normal coronal pulp tissue. (By courtesy of Professor R. Cawson.)

may not be formed if the blood supply is poor and it has been suggested that young teeth may form reactionary dentine more readily than old teeth for this reason. In addition, the severity of the stimulus may be relevant. A slowly progressing, small lesion may give time for a considerable reparative dentine response whereas with a more rapidly progressing lesion the response may be disorganized or even non-existent.

When formed, reactionary dentine provides extra protection for the odontoblasts and other cells of the pulp by increasing the distance between them and the injurious stimulus. In rather simple terms the pulp can be considered to be 'running away' and its retreat has important implications in the operative management of caries as will be seen in Chapter 10.

3.4.3. Inflammation of the Pulp

Inflammation is the fundamental response of all vascular connective tissues to injury. Inflammation of the pulp is called *pulpitis* and, as in any other tissue, it may be acute or chronic. The duration and intensity of the stimulus is partly responsible for the type of response. A low grade, long lasting stimulus may result in chronic inflammation whereas a sudden, severe stimulus is more likely to provoke an acute pulpitis.

In a slowly progressing carious lesion in dentine, the stimuli reaching the pulp are bacterial toxins and thermal and osmotic shocks from the external environment. The response to these low grade, sustained stimuli is chronic inflammation. However, once the organisms actually reach the pulp to create a 'carious exposure', acute inflammation is likely to supervene and be superimposed on the chronic inflammation.

Inflammatory reactions have vascular and cellular components. The cellular component is most obvious in chronic inflammation (*Fig.* 3.4) with lymphocytes, plasma cells, monocytes and macrophages all present within the tissue. In time there may be increased collagen production leading to fibrosis. These chronic inflammatory reactions may not endanger the vitality of the tooth.

Unfortunately, the same cannot be said of acute inflammation since in this process the vascular changes predominate, including dilatation of blood vessels, producing an initial acceleration of blood flow and fluid exudate. This exudate may later result in retardation of blood flow and vascular stasis. There is active emigration of neutrophils (*Fig.* 3.5) and all these factors contribute to an increase in tension of the tissue.

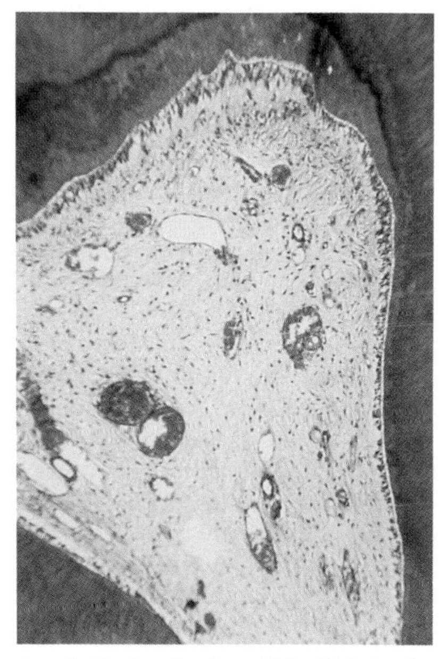

Fig. 3.5. Early acute pulpitis showing the widely dilated pulp vessels and early emigration of leucocytes. There is patchy oedema of the dying odontoblast layer. (By courtesy of Professor R. Cawson.)

The outcome of this process is often necrosis because the delicate connective tissue of the pulp is in a rigidly enclosed calcific chamber receiving its blood supply from a limited number of vessels passing through narrow root foramina. This has been thought to be due to the increase in pressure causing strangulation of the thin walled veins passing through the apical foramen. However, this may be an oversimplification of a more complex process.[2]

The sequel to pulpal necrosis is spread of inflammation into the periapical tissues (apical periodontitis). Once again, the inflammatory response may be acute or chronic.

3.4.4. Symptoms of Pulpitis

Many studies have attempted to correlate the symptoms of which a patient complains with the level of inflammation in the pulp as determined by histological examination. These correlations are poor and for this reason it is only possible to make some generalizations relating a patient's symptoms to the histological condition of the pulp.

The first of these generalizations is that a chronically inflamed pulp is usually symptomless. In contrast, acute inflammation is almost always painful, the painful response being initiated by hot, cold or sweet stimuli. Unfortunately the pain is often not well localized to the offending tooth and the patient may only be able to indicate which quadrant, or even which side of the mouth, is involved.

What matters to the clinician is whether or not the pulp is likely to survive, as a pulp that will die should be removed and the pulp canal sealed with an inert filling material (root canal filling) or the tooth should be extracted. Since clinical symptoms relate so poorly to pulp pathology there is an obvious problem here. A useful rule of thumb is to divide clinical pulpitis into *reversible pulpitis* and *irreversible pulpitis.*

In reversible pulpitis the clinician hopes to be able to preserve a healthy vital pulp. The clinical diagnosis of reversible pulpitis is made when the pain evoked by hot, cold or sweet stimuli is of short duration, disappearing when the stimulus is removed. On the other hand, if pain persists for minutes or hours after removal of the stimulus, a clinical diagnosis of irreversible pulpitis may be made and the pulp removed and replaced by a root filling. Alternatively, the tooth may be extracted.

Whereas acutely inflamed pulps are painful, necrotic pulps are painless since there are no viable nerves to transmit pain. However, once the periapical tissues are involved, another set of symptoms may develop. Chronic periapical inflammation is usually painless, but acute periapical inflammation is often very uncomfortable, the pain being well localized. The inflammatory exudate is sometimes sufficient to raise the tooth slightly in the socket. Such a tooth is tender to bite on and tender to touch because it acts as a piston in its socket transmitting forces directly to the inflamed periapical tissues. It is possible for acute periapical inflammation to become chronic and for chronic inflammation to become acute. The inflammation from acute periodontitis can spread to the adjacent soft tissues and produce a dramatic swelling. Eventually pus may discharge through a sinus and at this point pain is relieved and inflammation may then become chronic.

3.5. DEGENERATIVE OR DESTRUCTIVE CHANGES

The appearance of a carious lesion in dentine depends on the balance reached between the defence reactions already described and the destructive processes. The destructive processes include:

a. demineralization of dentine;
b. destruction of the organic matrix;
c. damage and death of the odontoblast;
d. pulpal inflammation proceeding to necrosis.

The pulp–dentine complex will often respond to the carious challenge before cavitation of the enamel, that is while the microorganisms are still confined to the tooth surface. This is particularly obvious in a slowly progressing lesion.

Once there is cavitation of enamel, bacteria can reach the dentine and the spectrum of defence reactions will be seen together with more marked destructive or degenerative changes.

3.6. HISTOLOGICAL APPEARANCE OF THE LESION BEFORE CAVITATION OF THE ENAMEL

Fig. 3.6 is a diagrammatic representation of a carious lesion developing on a smooth enamel surface. The four zones of enamel caries can be seen (translucent zone, dark zone, body of lesion and surface zone).

The advancing front of the enamel lesion has reached the enamel–dentine junction but the enamel surface is still intact. However, since the carious enamel is porous, acids, enzymes and other chemical stimuli from the tooth surface will reach the outer dentine evoking a response in the pulp–dentine complex. The defence reactions of reactionary dentine and translucent dentine may be seen together with some demineralization near the enamel–dentine junction.

Tubular sclerosis may obstruct the dentinal tubules causing their coronal ends to lose communication with the pulp. Therefore the tubules do not contain vital odontoblast processes and thus are 'dead tracts'. These tubules may contain gases, fluids and degenerating cell remnants *in vivo,* but in ground sections they become readily filled with air and appear dark or opaque in transmitted light.

3.7. HISTOLOGICAL APPEARANCE OF THE LESION AFTER CAVITATION OF THE ENAMEL

Once cavitation of the enamel occurs, bacteria have direct access to dentine and the tissue becomes infected. *Fig.* 3.7 is a diagrammatic representation of such a lesion. The three defence reactions of mild pulpal inflammation, reactionary dentine and tubular sclerosis can be seen. The sclerotic or

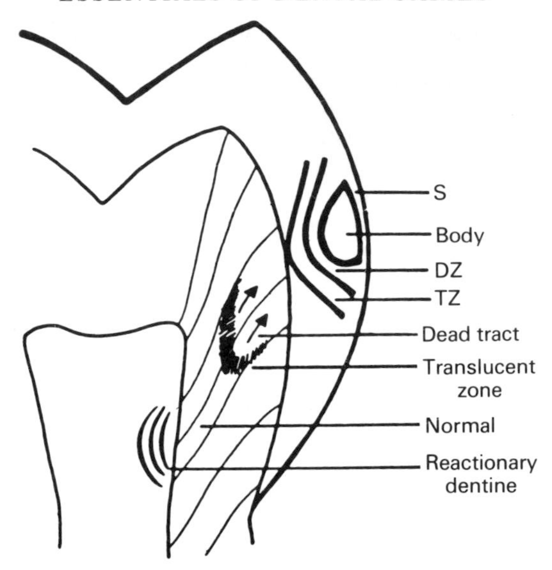

Fig. 3.6. Diagram of histological changes in enamel and dentine before cavitation of the enamel. (By courtesy of Professor N. W. Johnson.) S, Surface zone; Body, body of lesion; DZ, dark zone; TZ, translucent zone.

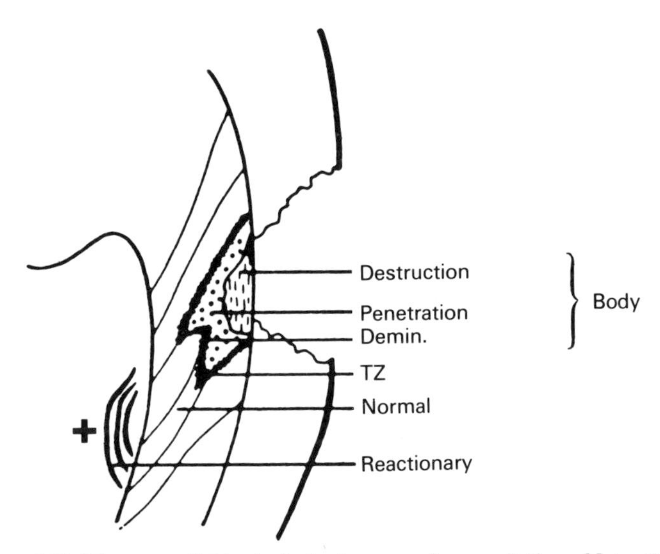

Fig. 3.7. Diagram of histological changes after cavitation. Note that demineralization of enamel precedes bacterial penetration. (By courtesy of Professor N. W. Johnson.) TZ, Translucent zone; DEMIN, demineralization.

translucent zone encloses the body of the lesion in dentine which may now be divided into three structural components. At the advancing edge is an area of *demineralized dentine* which does not yet contain bacteria. Superficial to this is a *zone of penetration,* so called because the tubules have become penetrated by microorganisms. Superficial to this is a *zone of destruction* or necrosis where microbial action has completely destroyed the substance of the dentine.

The fact that demineralization precedes bacterial penetration is of great importance in operative dentistry, particularly in deep cavities, since a major objective is to remove the infected and necrotic tissue and then place a therapeutic lining material over the demineralized dentine. The object of this is to kill any bacteria remaining, encourage remineralization of the residual dentine and the formation of reparative dentine. This operative procedure is called *indirect pulp capping* and will be discussed further in Chapter 10.

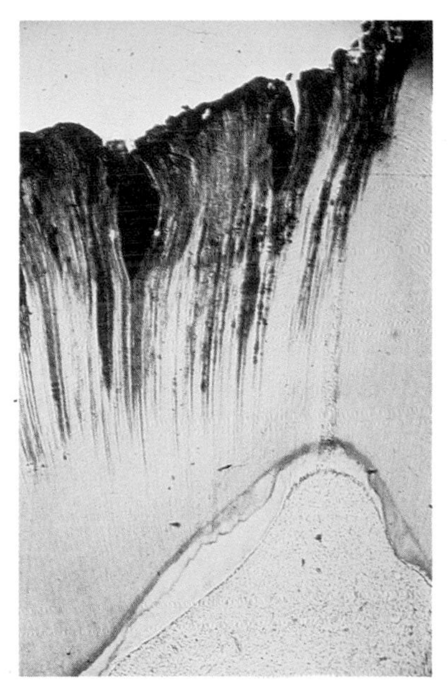

Fig. 3.8. Decalcified section of carious dentine showing dentinal tubules penetrated by deeply staining bacteria. In places the tubules appear to have been pushed apart by aggregations of bacteria called liquefaction foci. (By courtesy of Professor N. W. Johnson.)

Figs. 3.8 and 3.9 show some histological appearances of carious dentine. In *Fig.* 3.8 a decalcified section of carious dentine stained with haematoxylin and eosin shows the deeply staining bacteria streaming down the dentinal tubules. Aggregations of bacteria and necrotic tissue coalesce

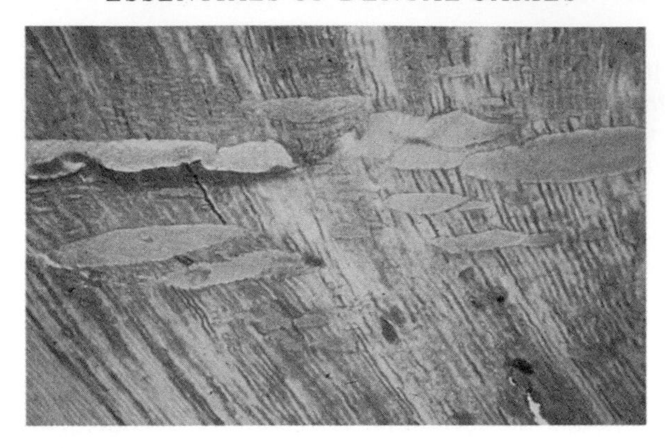

Fig. 3.9. Decalcified section of carious dentine showing tubules penetrated by bacteria. The tissue appears to have split at right angles to the tubules along the incremental lines of growth. These splits are called transverse clefts. (By courtesy of Professor N. W. Johnson.)

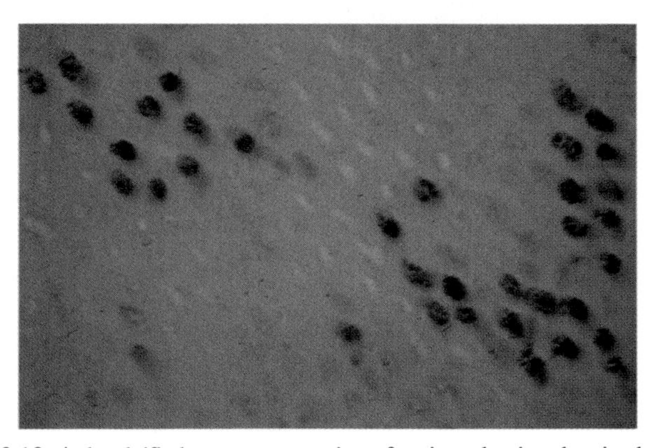

Fig. 3.10. A decalcified transverse section of carious dentine showing bacteria in the tubules. (By courtesy of Professor N. W. Johnson.)

to form *liquefaction foci* which appear to push the tubules apart. Destruction may also advance along the incremental lines of growth which are at right angles to the tubules to produce *transverse clefts* (*Fig.* 3.9).

In cross-section the bacteria can be seen in the tubules in *Fig.* 3.10 but in *Fig.* 3.11 destruction is more advanced and the bacteria are evident throughout the tissue.

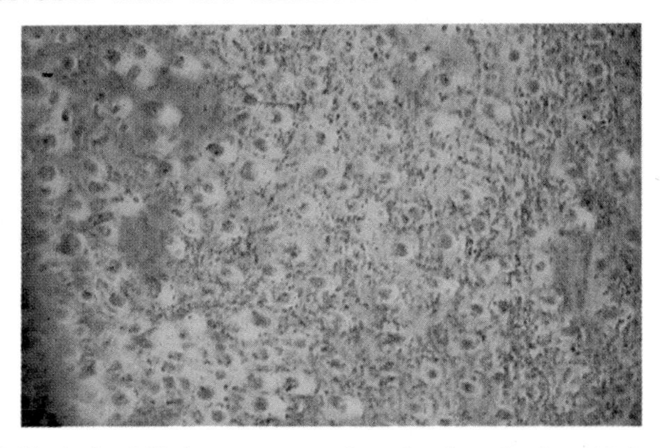

Fig. 3.11. A decalcified transverse section of carious dentine with bacteria evident throughout the tissue. (By courtesy of Professor N. W. Johnson.)

3.8. THE MICROBIOLOGY OF DENTINE CARIES

The first wave of bacteria infecting the dentine is primarily acidogenic. Since demineralization precedes bacterial penetration, the acid presumably diffuses ahead of the organisms. Lactobacilli are especially common, as are the cariogenic streptococci including *Streptococcus mutans.*

Towards the enamel–dentine junction there is a more mixed bacterial population, in which proteolytic and hydrolytic enzymes are added to the acid-producing organisms, resulting in destruction of the organic matrix of the tissue.

3.9. ACTIVE AND ARRESTED LESIONS

The rate of progress of caries in dentine is highly variable and under suitable environmental conditions the progress of the disease can be arrested and the lesion may even partly regress.

Clinically, actively progressing lesions are soft and light brown or yellow in colour. Because of the speed of development of the lesion the defence reactions will not be well developed. Pain is easily evoked by hot, cold and sweet stimuli. In contrast, arrested or slowly progressing lesions are dark brown in colour and have a hard, leathery consistency. Histologically the defence reactions of reparative dentine and tubular sclerosis are marked. The body of the lesion in dentine accumulates organic matter and mineral from oral fluids, the most striking remineralization taking place on and within the surface exposed to the oral environment.

It is very important to realize that even caries of dentine does not automatically progress. It is a dentist's responsibility to explain to patients how they may arrest the disease in their mouths.

3.10. ROOT CARIES[3]

Up to now this chapter has considered caries of dentine beneath enamel caries. However, in many mouths root surfaces become exposed and these surfaces are now susceptible to root caries and indeed appear more vulnerable to mechanical and chemical destruction then enamel.

Gingival recession is a prerequisite for exposure of a root surface, so it is hardly surprising that root caries is commonly seen in older people. It is associated with periodontal disease because this is a major cause of gingival recession. However, this does not mean that all patients with exposed root surfaces will automatically get root caries since a cariogenic plaque and a cariogenic diet are also required.

Clinically both active (soft, pale) and arrested or slowly progressing lesions (hard, dark brown) may be seen.

Early root surface lesions have been shown on microradiographs to be radiolucent zones (i.e. zones of demineralization) deep to a well mineralized surface layer which appears hypermineralized when compared to the neighbouring cementum. This hypermineralized surface zone covering early lesions is a consistent finding on exposed root surfaces but it is not present on non-exposed surfaces. This implies that mineral is likely to have precipitated from the saliva. Deep to the lesion there is frequently a hypermineralized area of tubular sclerosis.

Destruction of apatite crystals thus appears to take place deep to the surface before bacteria penetrate into the root cementum and dentine. In this respect enamel caries and root caries are similar. However, bacteria seem to penetrate into the tissue at an earlier stage in root caries than in coronal caries. The microorganisms invade the dentinal tubules and frequently spread in the less mineralized granular layer of Tomes. At this stage the overlying cementum frequently appears to separate along its incremental lines.

The recent dramatic decline in caries prevalence in children in many countries has resulted in an increased number of teeth being present in older individuals and for this reason root caries is of particular importance. Root caries is particularly difficult to treat by operative means and this will be discussed further in Chapter 10.

REFERENCES

1. Most of the information in this chapter has been derived from Silverstone L. M., Johnson N. W., Hardie J. M. and Williams R. A. D. (1984) *Dental Caries Aetiology, Pathology and Prevention.* London, Macmillan, Chapter 7.
2. Nicholls E. (1984) *Endodontics.* Bristol, Wright, Chapter 1.
3. Nyvad B. and Fejerskov O. (1982) Root surface caries: clinical, histopathological and microbiological features and clinical implications. *Int. Dent. J.* **32,** 311–326.

CHAPTER 4

DIAGNOSIS AND ITS RELEVANCE TO MANAGEMENT[1]

4.1. INTRODUCTION

The diagnosis of dental caries is fundamental to the practice of dentistry. This chapter will discuss the problems of diagnosis, concentrating on the so-called 'early' carious lesion. The word 'early' has been written in inverted commas because such a lesion may have been present in the mouth for many years in an arrested state (*see* Chapter 1.3; Chapter 2.1). An attempt will be made to answer four questions, namely:

a. Why is the diagnosis of caries in its 'early' stages important?
b. How can dental caries be diagnosed in its 'early' stages?
c. How can the patient 'at risk' to active caries be diagnosed?
d. What is the relevance of the diagnostic information to the management of the disease?

4.2. WHY IS THE DIAGNOSIS OF CARIES IN ITS 'EARLY' STAGES IMPORTANT?

Early diagnosis of the carious lesion has assumed a particular importance since it is now realized that dental caries can be arrested and remineralization can take place. Saliva is an excellent remineralizing fluid, particularly if it contains the fluoride ion. If the disease can be diagnosed in its earliest stages the balance can be tipped in favour of repair by use of fluoride, modifying diet and attempting to remove plaque (*see* Chapter 1, *Fig.* 1.12).

How early must the carious lesion be diagnosed in order to hope to be able to get it to repair? Obviously, small enamel lesions will partially remineralize more readily than large lesions. In addition, it has been shown that remineralized early carious lesions are actually more resistant to acid attack than sound enamel because they consist of larger crystals and contain more fluoride.

The next logical question is what is the 'point of no return' where we can no longer hope for remineralization or even arrest? At this point the restoration of damaged tissue by a filling material may be required. Perhaps the 'point of no return' is when a cavity is present, since a hole in the dental tissues is not expected to calcify up from the base. However, breaks in the enamel surface can partially remineralize, the base of the cavity becoming hard. Thus, one important question that the practitioner must answer is what will remineralize or arrest and what must be restored? In addition, is it possible to diagnose whether a cavity is present and of what relevance is this breach in the dental tissues?

4.3. HOW CAN DENTAL CARIES BE DIAGNOSED IN ITS 'EARLY' STAGES?

The diagnosis of caries in the surgery requires good lighting and dry, clean teeth. If heavy deposits of calculus or plaque are present the mouth should be cleaned before attempting accurate diagnosis. Each quadrant of the mouth is isolated with cotton wool rolls to prevent saliva wetting the teeth once they have been dried. Thorough drying should be carried out with a gentle blast of air from the three-in-one syringe.

Sharp eyes must be used to look for the earliest signs of disease. Traditionally, sharp probes have also been used to detect the 'tacky' feel of early cavitation. However, this approach should *not* be used because a sharp probe can actually damage an incipient carious lesion (*Fig.* 4.1) and by carrying microorganisms into the lesion may facilitate spread of caries.

Good bitewing radiographs are also essential in diagnosis. In this technique the central beam of X-rays is positioned to pass at right angles to the long axis of the tooth, and tangentially through the contact area. The

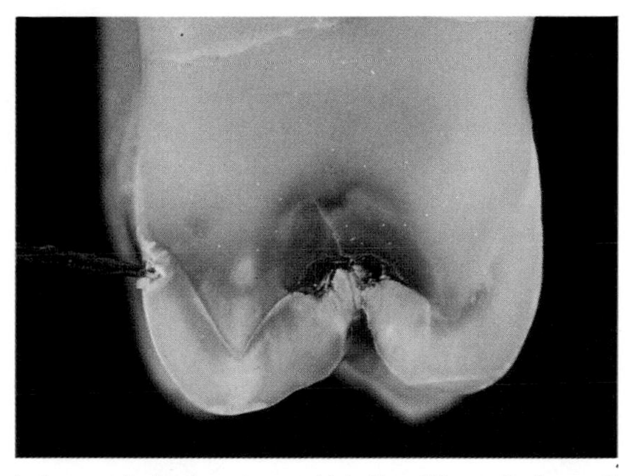

Fig. 4.1. A sharp probe has been jammed into the white spot lesion on the buccal aspect of this extracted molar. This picture shows the probe and the resulting damage. *Fig.* 3.2 shows this lesion before probing.

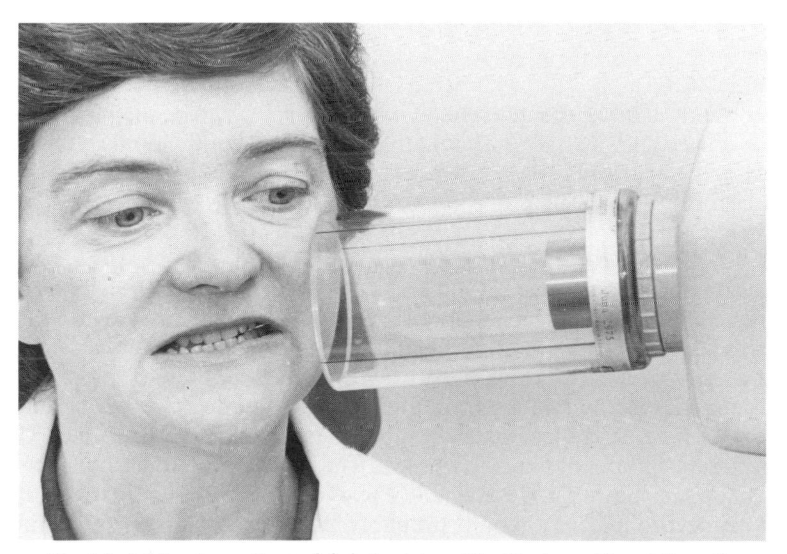

Fig. 4.2. A bitewing radiograph is being taken. The film is positioned lingually, the patient closing the teeth together to bite on a tab attached to the film.

film is positioned intraorally on the lingual side of the posterior teeth. Thc patient then closes the teeth together to bite on a tab attached to the film, thus holding it in position (*Fig.* 4.2). The type of radiograph resulting can be seen in *Fig.* 4.3.

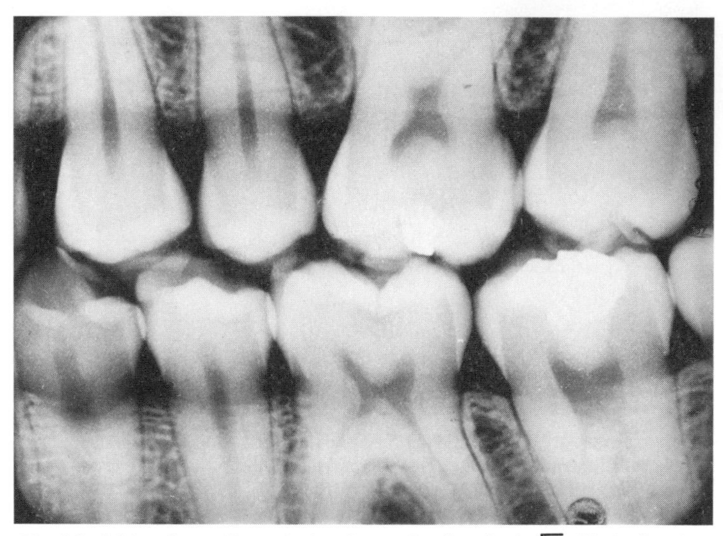

Fig. 4.3. A bitewing radiograph showing occlusal caries in ⌈6. Clinically, there was no detectable cavity in this tooth although the enamel was discoloured.

In order to answer the question of whether caries can be diagnosed in its 'early' stages and, if so, how should this be done, the individual sites where caries can occur must be considered separately. These are free smooth surfaces, pits and fissures and approximal surfaces.

4.3.1. Free Smooth Surfaces

Caries on free smooth enamel surfaces can be diagnosed with sharp eyes at the stage of the white or brown spot lesion (*Fig.* 1.5*c*) before cavitation has occurred, provided the teeth are clean, dry and well lit.

Root surface caries,[2] in its early stages, appears as one or more small, well defined, discoloured areas located along the cement–enamel junction (*Fig.* 4.4). The active lesions are yellowish or light brown in colour. They are softened without obvious cavitation. The arrested or slowly progressing lesions appear more darkly stained (*Fig.* 4.5), often almost black. If they were to be probed they would probably be softer than the surrounding normal cementum, but often their consistency seems more leathery than the active lesion. Frequently, however, dark passive lesions, even with cavitation, may be as hard as the non-diseased root surface or even harder. It must be emphasized that great care should be taken when using a probe on these lesions otherwise healing tissue may be damaged.

Root surface lesions tend to spread laterally and coalesce with minor neighbouring lesions and may thus eventually encircle the tooth. Commonly, the lesions extend only ½–1 mm in depth. They do not always

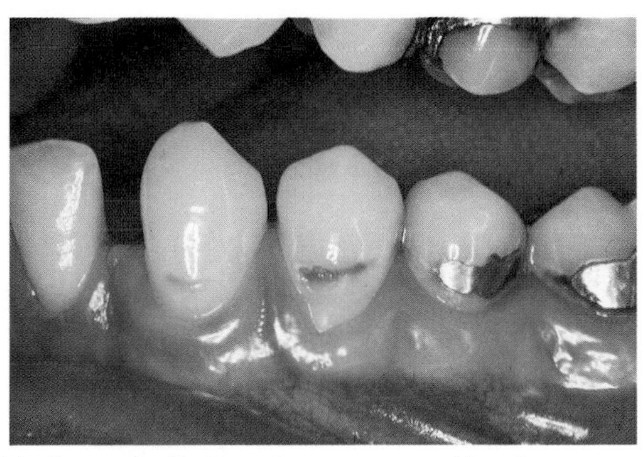

Fig. 4.4. Root surface caries at the cement–enamel junction.

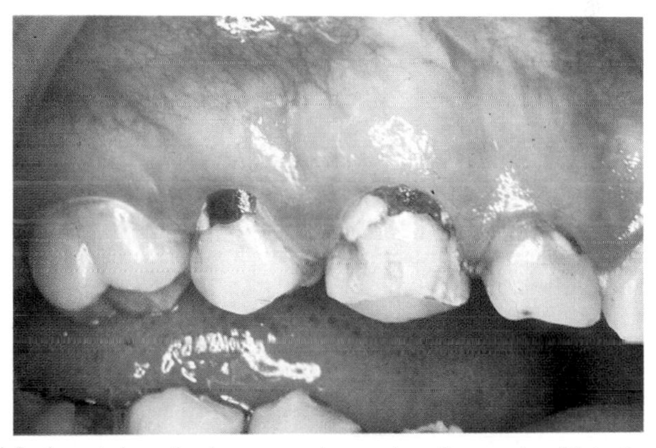

Fig. 4.5. Arrested or slowly progressing root surface caries. Note the dark staining.

spread apically as the gingival margin recedes but new lesions may develop later at the level of the new gingival margin. This may occur irrespective of an arrested lesion being located more coronally at the cement–enamel junction of the tooth.

4.3.2. Pits and Fissures

While caries on free, smooth surfaces is easy to see, caries in pits and fissures is difficult to diagnose at this early stage, since, histologically, the white spot lesions form on the walls of the fissure (*see* Chapter 2, *Fig.* 2.5). Thus the fissure which looks clinically caries-free may histologically show signs of early lesion formation. In addition, the fissure that is sticky to a

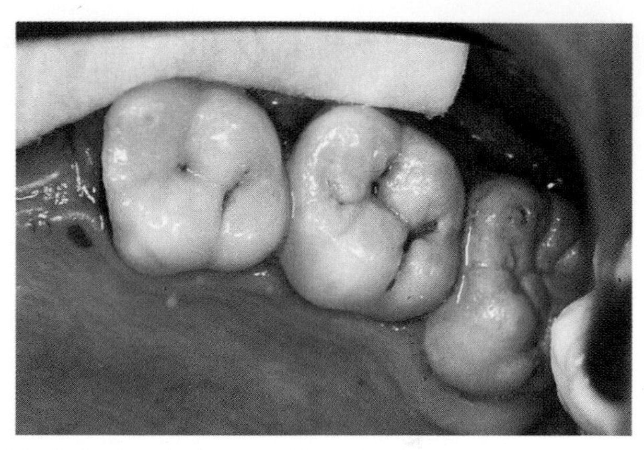

Fig. 4.6. Occlusal caries in upper first and second molars.

sharp probe may not be carious histologically. The stickiness may indicate fissure shape or the pressure exerted rather than caries and, indeed, a sharp probe can actually damage an incipient carious lesion. For these reasons it is suggested that the probe must be reserved for removing any plaque from the fissure to allow sharp eyes to pick up discolouration, cavitation and the grey appearance of enamel undermined by caries in the dentine beneath (*Figs.* 4.6 and 1.3).

In addition, bitewing radiographs are of great importance in the detection of occlusal caries, although by the time a lesion can be seen radiographically it is well into dentine (*Fig.* 4.3). Occlusal enamel may appear clinically caries-free or slightly discoloured with no cavity to be seen or probed, but a bitewing radiograph may show caries in dentine. Clinicians today are becoming very aware of the danger of missing occlusal caries and some would suggest that the pattern of disease is changing, with fluoride making the pits and fissures apparently hard and firm, while bitewings reveal radiolucency in the dentine beneath. It is interesting to speculate why the dentine should not remineralize in these cases. Perhaps there is a problem of access of salivary ions to the demineralized areas. It seems unlikely that such demineralized dentine is incapable of remineralization since the hard, stained appearance of remineralized root dentine is well known.

Thus, to summarize, it is difficult to diagnose caries in pits and fissures reliably in its earliest stages and the anatomy of the area may favour spread of the lesion rather than arrest. These facts are of considerable relevance in the management of the disease and will be discussed in Chapters 8 and 10.

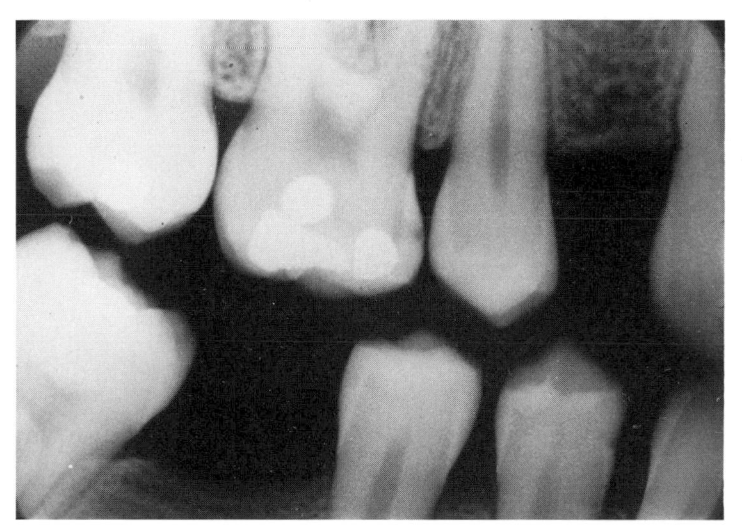

Fig. 4.7. A bitewing radiograph showing caries in enamel and dentine on the mesial aspect of the upper first molar. A lesion is also visible on the mesial aspect of the lower first premolar.

4.3.3. Approximal Surfaces

As with the fissure, it will be difficult to see the 'early' carious enamel lesion on an approximal surface. This is because the lesion forms just cervical to the contact area and vision is obscured by the adjacent tooth. The lesion is discovered visually at a relatively late stage when it has already progressed into dentine and is seen as a pinkish grey area shining up through the marginal ridge (*Fig.* 1.4). It must be emphasized again that the teeth should be isolated, clean and dry to see this.

In contrast, a root surface approximal lesion may be diagnosed visually but gingival health is mandatory for such diagnosis to be reliable. Thus, if the gingivae are red, swollen and tending to bleed, caries diagnosis in these areas should be deferred until scaling, polishing and improved oral hygiene have been instituted.

A sharp, curved probe (Briault) can be used gently to try to determine whether an approximal lesion is cavitated but if this instrument is used in a heavy-handed manner it can actually cause cavitation.

The bitewing radiograph is of paramount importance in the diagnosis of the approximal carious lesion (*Fig.* 4.7), although it should be remembered that the technique is relatively insensitive as it is not able to detect early subsurface demineralization. As shown diagrammatically in *Fig.* 4.8, the approximal enamel lesion appears as a dark triangular area in the enamel of the bitewing radiograph. The lesion may be in the outer enamel or be seen

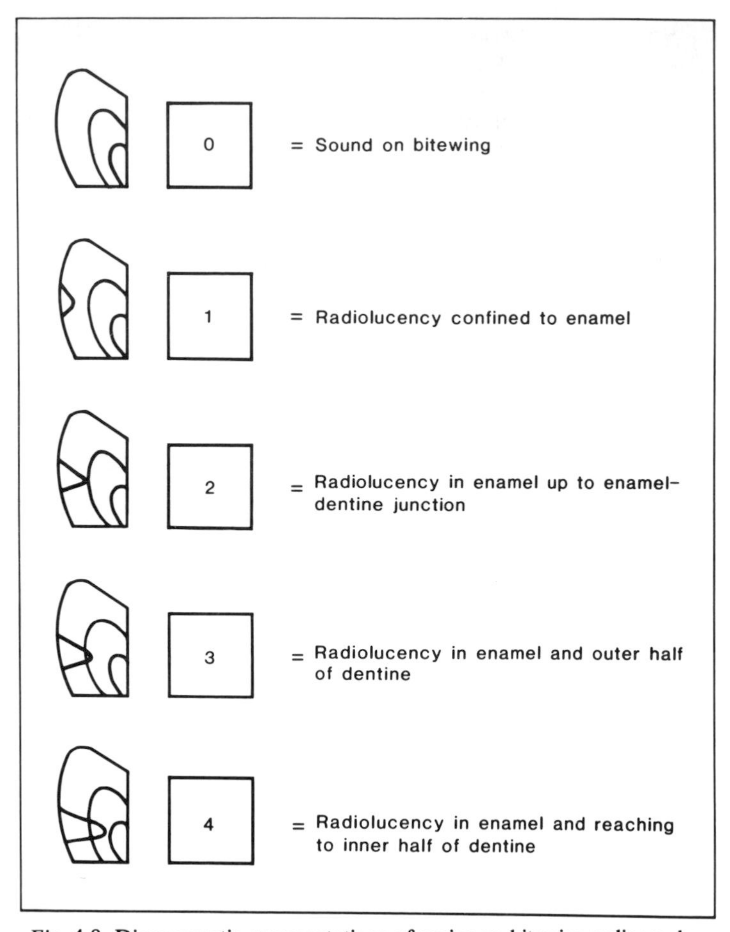

Fig. 4.8. Diagrammatic representations of caries on bitewing radiographs.

throughout the depth of the enamel. Larger lesions can be seen as a radiolucency in the enamel and outer half of dentine or as a radiolucency in the enamel reaching to the inner half of the dentine. The pulp is often exposed by the carious process in the latter instance.

Caries on the approximal root surface is also visible on a bitewing radiograph (*Fig.* 4.9) although this appearance is sometimes confused with the cervical radiolucency. The latter is a perfectly normal appearance caused by the absence of the dense enamel cap at the enamel–cement junction and absence of the interdental alveolar bone. Fortunately, root caries is visible clinically and a careful clinical re-examination will usually sort out any confusion.

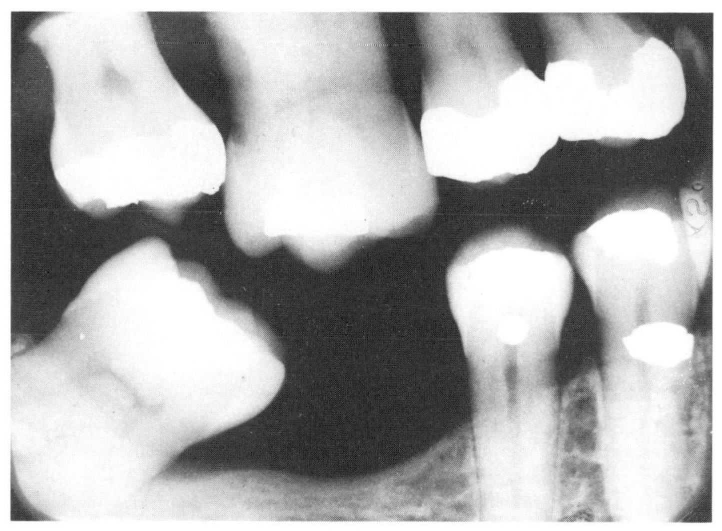

Fig. 4.9. A bitewing radiograph showing root caries on the distal aspect of the first upper molar. This tooth has overerupted following loss of the lower first molar.

It will be obvious that, to be of value, bitewing radiography must be carried out carefully. Overlapping contact points obscure what the clinician is trying to see and, unfortunately, slight differences in angulation of the film or X-ray beam will affect what is seen on the resultant radiograph. This is why the epidemiologist takes such care to take radiographs which are as reproducible as possible, using special film holders and standardizing exposure time and dose. In addition the epidemiologist will read the films dry, mounted and under standardized lighting conditions. Clinicians should take a note of this and avoid holding those dripping films to the sun!

Transmitted light can also be of considerable assistance in the diagnosis of approximal caries[3]. This technique consists of shining light through the contact point. A carious lesion has a lowered index of light transmission and therefore appears as a dark shadow that follows the outline of the decay through the dentine.

The technique has been used for many years in the diagnosis of approximal lesions in anterior teeth. Light is reflected through the teeth using the dental mirror and carious lesions are readily seen in the mirror (*Fig.* 4.10).

In posterior teeth a stronger light source is required and fibreoptic lights, with the beam reduced to 0·5 mm in diameter, have been used (*Fig.* 4.11). It is important that the diameter of the light source is small so that glare and loss of surface detail are eliminated. The light should be used with the teeth dry. This technique has particular advantages in patients with posterior

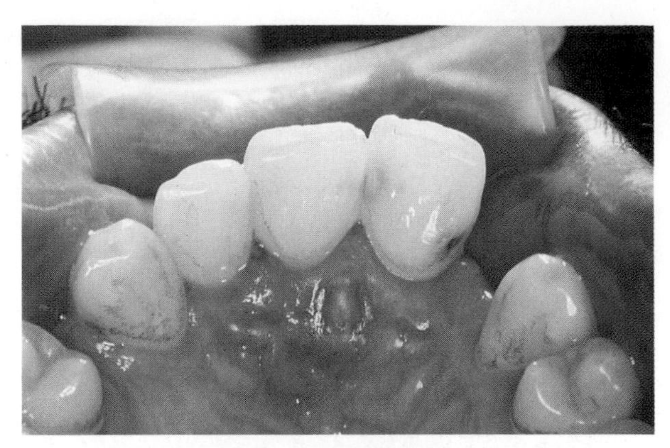

Fig. 4.10. A mirror view of the palatal aspect of the upper anterior teeth. Lesions are visible mesially and distally on the upper right central incisor.

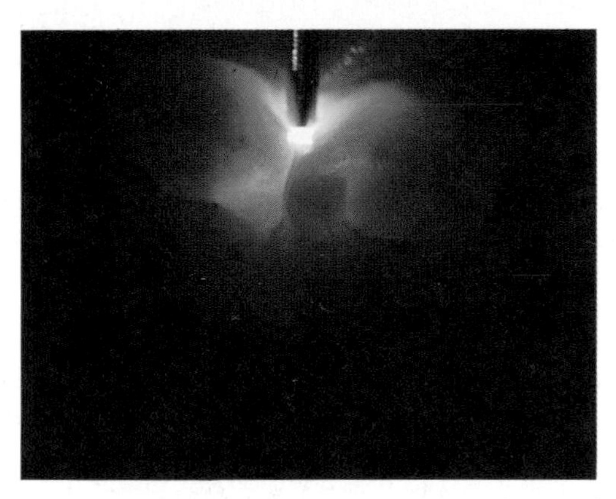

Fig. 4.11. Use of a fibreoptic light in the diagnosis of approximal caries. (By courtesy of Dr. C. Mitropoulos.)

crowding where bitewing radiographs will produce overlapping images and also in pregnant women where unnecessary radiation should be avoided.

4.4. HOW CAN THE PATIENT 'AT RISK' TO ACTIVE CARIES BE DIAGNOSED?[4]

It has already been stressed that caries should not be regarded purely as a process of demineralization but as an alternating process of destruction and repair. If the disease can be diagnosed early the dentist can help the patient institute preventive measures to tip the balance in favour of repair.

However, diagnosis implies more than just recording the number of cavities, their location and appearance. The dentist needs to know whether the patient is likely to develop new cavities and/or whether existing cavities are likely to progress.

This concept may be illustrated by two examples. Imagine examining a child of 5 years for the first time. The dentition appears caries-free. Does this patient need advice on prevention of disease or merely praise for doing so well? Now consider a 60-year-old patient, again seen for the first time; the mouth is fairly heavily restored and there is evidence of root caries on some teeth. Are these lesions likely to progress or have they already arrested? The dentist needs to know this before deciding how best to manage the patient.

Fortunately, it is possible to supplement the clinical examination by examining the diet and the saliva.

4.4.1. Repeated Clinical and Radiographic Examinations

The best assessment of caries risk is made from a detailed history, and clinical and radiographic examination. If there are numerous lesions, the patient is likely to be at risk. Even more information is gained if the dentist has the opportunity to examine the patient regularly, perhaps every 6 months, over a number of years. If no new lesions develop and existing 'early' lesions remain static and/or darken in colour, it can be concluded that caries risk is currently low.

The patient's age is also relevant to caries risk. Caries occurs most frequently in young people. Once susceptible sites, such as fissures and approximal surfaces, have been restored, the caries rate is reduced in many mouths. However, clinicians should not be lulled into a false sense of security by this generalization because older people can certainly develop new carious lesions if such factors as diet or salivary flow are altered.

4.4.2. Dietary History

As diet is one of the main factors in the development of dental caries, a dietary assessment is a fundamental part of the examination and should always be done in patients with a high caries activity. The various techniques of diet analysis will be discussed in detail in Chapter 6.

4.4.3. Salivary Secretion Rate and Buffer Capacity

Saliva is a protective fluid as far as the mouth is concerned. A low secretion rate and a low buffer capacity lead to reduced elimination of microorganisms and food remnants, impaired neutralization of acids and a reduced ability to remineralize the early enamel lesion. A low salivary secretion rate may be accompanied by an increased number of *Streptococcus mutans* and lactobacilli. Thus increased caries activity may be seen in persons with a reduced salivary secretion rate. This will be discussed in more detail in Chapter 5.

Stimulated salivary secretion rate can be determined by asking the patient to hold a piece of paraffin wax in the mouth until it becomes soft; the saliva produced during this time is swallowed. Once the patient can chew comfortably on the wax he should be asked to expectorate all saliva formed over a 5-minute period into a suitable measuring cylinder. The volume of saliva secreted is measured and the secretion rate expressed in millilitres per minute.

Normal stimulated secretion rate in adults	1–2 ml per min
Low stimulated secretion rate in adults	<0·7 ml per min
Severely dry mouth	<0·1 ml per min

Some of the paraffin-stimulated saliva can now be used to give an indication of the buffering capacity. Since the buffering capacity of saliva generally increases after eating, it is preferable to collect samples about two hours after a meal.

Three millilitres of 0·005 mol/l HCl solution is added to 1 ml of saliva. The sample is shaken and the stopper removed to eliminate carbon dioxide. The sample is allowed to stand for 10 minutes and then the final pH is measured with pH indicator paper or a pH meter. Special kits are commercially available (Dento-buff) which are convenient for chairside use. These contain a small vial with a weak acid and a colour indicator. The kit also holds a syringe with which 1 ml of the saliva sample can be injected into the test vial. After mixing, the resulting colour is compared with an accompanying colour chart.

Normal buffering capacity	final pH 5–7
Low buffering capacity	final pH 4

If salivary examination shows low values for secretion rate and buffering capacity, tests should be repeated to determine whether the values are occasional or constant. If they are constant, the causative factor has to be determined (Chapter 5).

4.4.4. Microbiological Examination

Some microorganisms are more important than others in the pathogenesis of dental caries. There is now some evidence that individuals with a high level of *S. mutans* infection may be at risk to dental caries. In addition, there is some evidence that a high level of lactobacilli is associated with a cariogenic diet. High levels of this organism are also associated with multiple open cavities and such cavities should be excavated and temporarily dressed (Chapter 10) before determining the level of lactobacillus infection.

Streptococcus mutans and lactobacillus counts can be carried out on paraffin stimulated saliva. The saliva sample is collected and some of it is transferred to a transport vial, containing a transport fluid, using a syringe or pipette.

The sample is then transferred to the laboratory where it is homogenized, diluted quantitatively and cultivated on selective media for *S. mutans* and lactobacilli. In most laboratories *S. mutans* is cultivated on mitis salivarius agar containing sucrose and bacitracin. For cultivation of lactobacilli, SL-agar is generally used. The number of typical colonies at a suitable dilution is counted and the figure obtained is multiplied by the dilution factor. This gives the number of *S. mutans* and lactobacilli respectively for each millilitre of saliva.

High value	>1 000 000 *S. mutans*	>100 000 lactobacilli
Low value	<100 000 *S. mutans*	<1 000 lactobacilli

A commercially available kit (Dento-cult) is available for lactobacillus counts and a similar kit has been developed for *S. mutans* counts. This may make it feasible for these tests to be carried out in the surgery.

4.4.5. Assessment of Findings

For assessment of the actual caries risk information from the case history, the clinical and radiographic examination, the dietary history and the salivary tests all have to be considered. No single negative factor should be taken to imply a high caries risk. Although sugar consumption and the number of *S. mutans* are closely associated with caries, there are many people with high *S. mutans* counts who do not develop caries. Similarly, some people can eat sugar frequently but be caries-free. Caries is a disease caused by several factors, and must be treated as such.

4.5. THE RELEVANCE OF THE DIAGNOSTIC INFORMATION TO THE MANAGEMENT OF THE DISEASE[1,5]

It is important to remember that clinical and radiographic diagnoses may be inaccurate. No one can be sure of recording the same caries diagnosis on different occasions on one patient; to prove the point the student might like to collect a number of bitewing radiographs, note their findings and then repeat the examinations a week later. Students will find they are not consistent with themselves, let alone a colleague. However, they should not feel too despondent about this since the trained epidemiologist is only 70–80 per cent reliable! When the disease is at an early stage, diagnoses are more likely to be incorrect.

When caries is diagnosed the clinician must decide how the disease should be treated. Currently there are two possible approaches:

a. To use preventive measures to attempt to arrest the disease.

b. Surgically to remove and replace the damaged tissues and prevent recurrence.

These two approaches will now be considered in the light of the diagnostic information available.

4.5.1. Free, Smooth Surfaces

Caries on free, smooth surfaces can be diagnosed at the stage of the white spot lesion, that is before cavitation occurs. However, on the first occasion dentist and patient meet, it may not be obvious whether such a lesion represents active decay or a chronic static lesion which has been present for many years. Thus although it is easy to diagnose it may not be easy to interpret. The wise practitioner will probably discuss the problem with the patient, carry out diet analysis and carry out laboratory tests if such facilities are available. Preventive measures such as dietary advice (Chapter 6), use of fluoride (Chapter 7), and improved plaque control (Chapter 9) can then be instituted and the lesion reassessed in 6 months.

4.5.2. Pits and Fissures

Since caries in pits and fissures is difficult to diagnose in its earliest stage and since fissures are particularly susceptible sites, the dentist may decide to fissure seal susceptible teeth as soon after eruption as possible. Fissure sealants are materials which cover and protect the fissure and are discussed in detail in Chapter 8.

The occlusal lesion which shows on a bitewing radiograph (*Fig.* 4.3) should be restored (*see* Chapter 10). A small occlusal restoration, carefully executed, is preferable to the risk of waiting until an exposure necessitates root canal therapy. The anatomy of the fissure and the consequent shape of the carious lesion often results in gross undermining of enamel by the carious process. In addition, epidemiological work has shown that whereas an approximal lesion may develop slowly, taking three to four years to reach dentine, the rate of progress of initial pit and fissure caries is more rapid, cavitation occurring in less than 1 year up to the age of 13 years. For these reasons the authors currently treat fissure caries less conservatively than smooth surface caries, being more inclined to restore and prevent recurrence, than to rely on preventive measures alone.

4.5.3. Approximal Surfaces

The decision to cut a cavity or treat with preventive measures only can be particularly difficult on approximal surfaces. The decision is difficult because it is still not clear what the radiographic picture means clinically. Despite this, today's clinician must have some guidelines as to when to restore and thus positive suggestions will be given in this section.

In epidemiological studies, ranking systems are used which divide enamel and dentine into inner and outer halves so that a more sensitive indication of lesion depth is possible. One such system is illustrated in *Fig.* 4.8 and will be used to discuss the clinical problem of when to restore. There will be no argument at the two ends of the spectrum. Teeth that are sound on the radiograph will be left alone, although it must still be remembered that early white spots may still be present, the radiographic technique being less sensitive than the naked eye. Teeth that are shown to be very carious on the radiograph will be restored and measures instituted to prevent recurrence. However, the decisions are less clear cut when the radiographic appearances 1, 2 and 3 are considered.

If the nick apparent in outer enamel on the bitewing radiograph is considered (no. 1, *Fig.* 4.8), there is histological evidence to show that the lesion is larger than it looks on the radiograph. It is also known that approximal caries is a relatively slow disease which may take some two to four years to progress through the enamel of permanent teeth. In addition dentists must remember their fallibility in diagnosis because the lesions they think they see on bitewing radiographs may not be present.

For all these reasons the early nick in outer enamel seen on a bitewing radiograph should be given a chance to arrest by instituting preventive measures, particularly as there is now some evidence that the early lesion may be more resistant to further acid attack than sound enamel.

Although there are several studies on the rate at which caries progresses through enamel in permanent teeth (0–2 on scale, *Fig.* 4.8), there appears to be no information on the speed of progress through dentine (2–4 on scale, *Fig.* 4.8). This is an important piece of information which the profession currently does not have.

In addition, it is not known whether there is a break in the enamel surface (cavitation) when a lesion is seen on a bitewing radiograph. However, it is known that cavities will not 'fill up from the bottom' and cavitation is a point of no return as far as remineralization is concerned although such a lesion might arrest. A cavity will certainly be a plaque trap unless it is accessible to a toothbrush filament but it could be argued that, if diet is corrected, minor breaks in the outer enamel are of little consequence.

The state of our ignorance on the interpretation of the approximal lesion seen on a bitewing radiograph could be summarized thus:

a. the lesion is histologically larger than it looks;

b. it is not known whether there is a cavity, although it has been shown that the higher the patient's caries prevalence, the more likely the lesion is to be cavitated;

c. the average time for lesions to remain confined to the enamel is three to four years in permanent teeth;

d. the time taken to pass through dentine is not known;

e. the lesion can partially remineralize;

f. it is not known if the lesion can completely remineralize and disappear on a radiograph;

g. it is not known, unless reproducible serial radiographs are available, whether a lesion shown on a bitewing radiograph represents active decay or a chronic static lesion that has already arrested.

Whether to cut or attempt to arrest the lesion which on the radiograph is through enamel and just in to dentine is a difficult clinical decision, particularly at the present time when the profession is not sure that the apparent decline in dental caries will be accompanied by a slowing of the disease process. When caries has apparently penetrated enamel on the radiograph (2 on scale, *Fig.* 4.8), the authors would treat preventively and reassess in 6 months. However, once dentine is involved radiographically (3 on scale, *Fig.* 4.8), operative treatment is indicated unless serial radiographs indicate that the lesion is static and has been present for many years. However, these rules should not be rigid because every clinician knows that caries prevalence and rate of progress of the disease varies enormously from patient to patient. A combination of history, examination, diet analysis and salivary tests will obviously assist in identifying those patients at particular risk.

4.5.4. Root Caries

Early diagnosis of root caries is of particular clinical importance because advanced disease is virtually impossible to treat by operative means. Lesions coalesce to encircle the neck of the tooth and eventually the crown may break off.

Previous root surface caries experience and salivary flow rate have been shown to be good predictors of root caries risk. A combination of dietary control, use of topical fluorides and meticulous plaque control should be used to prevent the development of new lesions.

By using such an approach it may be possible to reharden even rather extensive root caries. In this connection it should be remembered that although the lesions may be extensive, they are usually shallow. As the lesions become arrested, a brownish black discolouration cannot be avoided, and there may also be slight cavitation. However, a black, concave, hard area on a tooth may be preferable to a deteriorating restoration which is difficult to keep clean and where caries is likely to develop along the faulty margins. Vigorous probing of root carious lesions should be avoided so as not to impair the surface of the tooth.

4.5.5. Deciduous Teeth

The majority of material written about the diagnosis and management of caries in the permanent dentition is applicable to the deciduous dentition. For instance, it is just as important to use bitewing radiographs for diagnosis of caries in deciduous teeth as in permanent teeth.

However, there are some obvious differences which are worth stressing:

a. Deciduous teeth do not usually develop root caries unless they are retained into adult life when their roots may become exposed and therefore vulnerable.

b. Deciduous teeth are smaller than permanent teeth. The pulps are relatively large in proportion to the enamel and dentine.

c. For this reason the disease may pass through enamel and dentine and affect the pulp more rapidly than in the permanent dentition.

d. Thus the caries-susceptible child should be examined frequently and operative intervention may be advisable earlier than in the permanent dentition.

e. Finally, since deciduous teeth are small, operative dentistry may be difficult if lesions are too large. For this reason many paediatric dentists would advise operative treatment of approximal lesions which have just reached the enamel–dentine junction.

REFERENCES

1. Kidd E. A. M. (1984) The diagnosis and management of the 'early' carious lesion in permanent teeth. *Dent. Update* **11,** 69–81.
2. Nyvad B. and Fejerskov O. (1982) Root surface caries: clinical, histopathological and microbiological features and clinical implications. *Int. Dent. J.* **32,** 311–326.
3. Mitropoulos C. M. (1985) A comparison of fibreoptic transillumination with bitewing radiographs. *Br. Dent. J.* **159,** 21–23.
4. Krasse B. (1985) *Caries Risk. A Practical Guide for Assessment and Control.* Chicago, Quintessence.
5. Elderton R. J. (1985) Assessment and clinical management of early caries in young adults: invasive versus non-invasive methods. *Br. Dent. J.* **158,** 440–444.

CHAPTER 5

SALIVA AND CARIES

5.1. INTRODUCTION

Saliva is a complex oral fluid consisting of a mixture of secretions from the major salivary glands and the minor glands of the oral mucosa. About 90 per cent of the total salivary flow is from the parotid and submaxillary glands, 5 per cent from the sublingual and 5 per cent from the minor salivary glands. Most of this saliva (90 per cent) is produced at mealtimes as a response to stimulation due to tasting and chewing. For the rest of the day, although salivary flow is low, it is extremely important. In healthy individuals the teeth are constantly bathed by up to 0·5 ml of 'resting saliva' which helps to protect the teeth, tongue and mucous membranes of the mouth and oropharynx. Salivation virtually stops during sleep because the salivary glands do not secrete spontaneously in the human.

The normal *stimulated* secretion rate in adults is 1–2 ml per minute. However, it may be reduced to less than 0·1 ml per minute in individuals with severe salivary gland malfunction. The terms 'xerostomia' (Greek: xeros = dry; stoma = mouth) and 'dry mouth' are used to describe this condition. In less severe cases of hyposalivation the secretion rate is between 0·7 and 0·1 ml per minute.

5.2. SALIVA AND DENTAL HEALTH[1, 2, 3]

5.2.1. Functions of Saliva

Although saliva aids swallowing and digestion, and is required for optimal function of the taste buds, its most important role is to maintain the integrity of the teeth, tongue and mucous membranes of the oral and oral-pharyngeal regions. Its protective action is manifested in several ways:

a. It forms a protective mucoid coating on the mucous membrane which acts as a barrier to irritants and prevents desiccation.

b. Its flow helps to clear the mouth of food, cellular and bacterial debris and consequently retards plaque formation.

c. It is capable of regulating the pH of the oral cavity by virtue of its bicarbonate content as well as its phosphate and amphoteric protein constituents. An increase in secretion rate usually results in an increase in pH and buffering capacity. The mucous membrane is thus protected from acid in food or vomit. In addition the fall in plaque pH, as a result of the action of acidogenic organisms, is minimized.

d. It helps to maintain the integrity of teeth in several ways because of its calcium and phosphate content. It provides minerals which are taken up by the incompletely formed enamel surface soon after eruption (post-eruptive maturation). Tooth dissolution is prevented or retarded and remineralization is enhanced by the presence of a copious salivary flow. The film of glycoprotein formed on the tooth surface by saliva (the acquired pellicle) may also protect the tooth by reducing wear due to erosion and abrasion.

e. Saliva is capable of considerable antibacterial and antiviral activity by virtue of its content of specific antibodies (secretory IgA) as well as lysozyme, lactoferrin and lactoperoxidase.

5.2.2. Causes of Reduced Salivary Flow

There are numerous systemic conditions (listed in *Table* 5.1) which can alter salivary flow rate. The most serious causes of malfunction of the salivary glands are radiotherapy in the region of these glands, drugs and disease.

Table 5.1 Systemic Causes of 'Dry Mouth'

Drugs
Psychological factors
Sjögren's syndrome
Hormonal changes (post-menopause)
Diabetes mellitus
Neurological diseases
Pancreatic disturbances
Liver disturbances
Nutritional deficiencies
Systemic lupus erythematosus
? Ageing

Radiotherapy

The exposure of the salivary glands to radiation during radiotherapy for neoplasms in the head and neck region usually results in a severe reduction in salivary flow (less than 0·1 ml/min). Associated with the marked reduction in salivary flow there is a considerable increase in its total protein content resulting in a thick viscous secretion which makes the condition even more uncomfortable. The time taken for salivary flow rate to return towards normal values varies and depends on the individual as well as the dose to which the glands have been exposed. Thus, in some patients, there is a considerable improvement after three months while in others xerostomia may be permanent as a result of atrophy of the glands induced by the radiation.

Drugs

A large number of therapeutic drugs affect salivary flow rate as well as its composition. Listed in *Table* 5.2 are the groups of drugs which result in decreased flow. Consequently, if any of them are used for more than a few weeks, steps must be taken to protect the teeth from caries.

In addition, chemotherapy with cytotoxic drugs used in the management of some malignancies may also cause acute onset of dry mouth.

Table 5.2 Medications which retard salivary flow

Antidepressants
Antipsychotic drugs
Tranquillizers
Hypnotics
Antihistamines
Anticholinergics
Antihypertensives
Diuretics
Anti-Parkinsonian drugs
Appetite suppressants

Disease

Acute and chronic inflammation of the salivary glands (sialadenitis), benign or malignant tumours as well as Sjögren's syndrome, may all lead to xerostomia depriving the individual of the protective action of saliva. Sjögren's syndrome is an autoimmune connective tissue disorder. Principally it affects the salivary and lacrymal glands which become damaged by lymphocytic infiltrates and therefore produce less secretion. Fifteen to 30 per cent of patients with rheumatoid arthritis also have Sjögren's syndrome. For this reason the possibility of a dry mouth should be considered in patients with rheumatoid arthritis.

Age

It is generally assumed that a reduction in salivary flow is the inevitable result of ageing. However, recent studies show that, at least for the parotid gland flow, there is no diminution of stimulated fluid output with increasing age in healthy subjects not taking therapeutic drugs. On the other hand, there is some evidence that atrophic changes occur in submandibular glands with age, resulting in reduced flow and small changes in composition of the saliva. It would seem, therefore, that any small decrease in salivary flow as a result of ageing is slight compared with reductions in flow due to disease and the use of drugs in this group of individuals.

5.2.3. General Consequences of Reduced Salivary Flow

The useful role of saliva is not usually appreciated until there is a shortage. The contribution that saliva makes to oral health is therefore best demonstrated by examining the consequences of xerostomia. The oral mucosa, without the lubricating and protective action of saliva, is more prone to traumatic ulceration and infection. Mucositis presents as tenderness, pain or a burning sensation and is exacerbated by spicy foods, fruits, alcoholic and carbonated beverages, hot drinks and tobacco. Taste sensation is altered and chewing and swallowing present difficulties, particularly if the food is bulky or dry. When salivary flow is diminished foods requiring a great deal of chewing are not well tolerated. Since chewing itself helps to stimulate salivary flow, the condition is exacerbated even if there is some glandular activity left. Speaking may become difficult because of lack of lubrication. These individuals also suffer from extreme sensitivity of teeth to heat and cold, especially if any dentine is exposed. Edentulous patients may have problems tolerating dentures, probably because of reduction in surface tension between the dry mucosa and the fitting surface of the denture.

There is an increase in dental plaque accumulation and a modification of the plaque flora in favour of candida, *Streptococcus mutans* and lactobaccillus. Consequently, in patients with dry mouths, candidal infections and gingivitis are frequent and rampant caries is common if no preventive measures are taken. 'Radiation caries' will be discussed in detail later (*see* section 5.4.2).

5.3. AMELIORATION OF 'DRY MOUTH'

5.3.1. Salivary Stimulants

Salivary stimulants will only be helpful when there is some glandular activity present. The following agents have been used:

a. Chewing gum or sucking acidic sweets may increase salivary flow. However, if a patient is dentate, gum may be very damaging to the teeth unless it is sucrose-free. It is also not advisable to recommend fruit drops flavoured with artificial sweeteners normally marketed for diabetics since some of these are very acidic and may indeed dissolve enamel and dentine. Some patients benefit from chewing a piece of paraffin wax (1·0–1·5 mg) three to five times a day and prefer this to flavoured chewing gum.

b. Two products—Mouth Lubricant and Lemon Mucilage—which are available from hospital pharmacies, contain citric acid and have a pH of 2·0 and 2·8 respectively. It is not surprising that both these solutions are very damaging to enamel and dentine. Although they may be suitable for edentulous patients, they should never be prescribed for dentate individuals.

c. Salivix is a proprietary lozenge containing malic acid, gum arabic, calcium lactate, sodium phosphate, lycasin and sorbitol. The manufacturers claim that it stimulates salivary flow and that, because of the calcium lactate buffer present, it does not demineralize enamel in spite of a pH of 4·0. However, since it has not been tested on dentine, more work is required before it can be recommended for dentate patients.

d. The systemic use of drugs such as pilocarpine hydrochloride and nicotinic acid has proved successful in stimulating saliva in some cases. However, their use is not recommended because of unpleasant side effects.

5.3.2. Saliva Substitutes

In the past, individuals with 'dry mouth' have had to rely on frequent moistening with water or liquids such as liquid paraffin or glycerine. Several saliva substitutes are now available to make the patient feel more comfortable and ideally to supply calcium and phosphate ions to aid remineralization. Saliva substitutes have been produced in the form of a solution, spray or lozenge.

Solutions

a. Hypromellose (pH 8·0) is a combination of the artificial tear preparation hydroxypropyl-methyl cellulose with saccharine.

b. V.A. Oralube (pH 7·0) is the saliva substitute formulated in the Veteran's Administration Hospital in Texas to simulate the viscosity and electrolyte levels of whole saliva.[4] It contains sodium fluoride as well as calcium, phosphate, potassium and magnesium ions and methyl cellulose (*see Table* 5.3) and is designed specifically to remineralize enamel and dentine. Patient acceptability has been tested and found to be good. A product, called Luborant, is based on this formulation and is commercially available through Antigen International Ltd.

Sprays

a. Saliva Orthana (pH 7·0) (Nycomed, UK Ltd) is a proprietary preparation in the form of a spray. It is unique because besides sodium fluoride, calcium, phosphate, sodium, magnesium and potassium ions, it contains mucin instead of carboxymethyl cellulose to provide viscosity.[5] The mucin is extracted from the gastric mucosa of the pig.

Table 5.3 Formulation for V.A. Oral Lubricant

Sodium carboxymethyl cellulose	40·0 g
Potassium chloride	2·498 g
Sodium chloride	3·462 g
Magnesium chloride ($6H_2O$)	0·235 g
Calcium chloride ($2H_2O$)	0·665 g
Dipotassium hydrogen orthophosphate	3·213 g
Potassium dihydrogen orthophosphate	1·304 g
Sodium fluoride	17·68 mg
Methyl *p*-hydroxybenzoate	8·0 g
70 per cent sorbitol	171·0 g
Flavouring and colouring agents as desired	
Water	ad 4 000 ml

The hydrophilic high molecular weight glycoproteins present in mucin bind water, decrease surface tension and so, theoretically, provide an ideal protective layer for both the teeth and the epithelial membranes. Although patient acceptability has been tested and found to be good, it has not been compared adequately with any similar product containing carboxymethyl cellulose instead of mucin.

b. Glandosane (pH 5·1) (Dylade Company Ltd) is similar in composition to Saliva Orthana except that it does not contain fluoride and is formulated with hydroxymethyl cellulose instead of mucin. However, its pH is somewhat lower because it contains carbon dioxide as a propellant for the spray. It should not, therefore, be used for dentate patients.

Lozenges

Polyox is a lozenge containing polyethelene oxide which exhibits similar viscoelastic properties to saliva when dissolved in the mouth. Patients have found it acceptable only if there is enough saliva present in which to dissolve the lozenge. However, a 1 or 2 per cent solution has been found to be very helpful on the fitting surface of dentures.[6]

Unfortunately, there have been few controlled studies to date comparing the acceptability and effectiveness of these preparations so that no particular substitute for saliva can be recommended. However, it is obvious that any preparation with a low pH should never be used for dentate patients. Ideally, the saliva substitute should either contain fluoride or be supplemented by a daily fluoride mouthwash (*see* section 5.4.3).

5.4. SALIVA AND CARIES

5.4.1. Anti-cariogenic Actions of Saliva

Theoretically saliva can influence the carious process in several ways:

a. The flow of saliva can reduce plaque accumulation on the tooth surface and also increase the rate of carbohydrate clearance from the oral cavity.

b. The diffusion into plaque of salivary components such as calcium, phosphate, hydroxyl and fluoride ions can reduce the solubility of enamel and promote remineralization of early carious lesions.

c. The carbonic acid–bicarbonate buffering system, as well as ammonia and urea constituents of the saliva, can buffer and neutralize the pH fall which occurs when plaque bacteria metabolize sugar. The pH and buffering capacity of saliva is related to its secretion rate. The pH of parotid saliva increases from about 5·5 for unstimulated saliva to about 7·4 when the flow rate is high. The respective pH values for submandibular saliva are 6·4 and 7·1. An increase in the secretion rate of saliva also results in a greater buffering capacity. In both cases this is due to the increase in sodium and bicarbonate concentrations.

d. Several non-immunological components of saliva such as lysozyme, lactoperoxidase and lactoferrin have a direct antibacterial action on plaque microflora or may affect their metabolism so that they become less acidogenic.

e. Immunoglobulin A (IgA) molecules are secreted by plasma cells within the salivary glands, while another protein component is produced in the epithelial cells lining the ducts. The total concentration of IgA in saliva may be inversely related to caries experience.

f. Salivary proteins could increase the thickness of the acquired pellicle and so help to retard the movement of calcium and phosphate ions out of enamel.

Whilst there is no doubt that saliva possesses all the anti-caries properties listed above, research workers have been frustrated in their attempts to relate directly any particular salivary factor to the incidence of caries. One of the reasons for their failure is the fact that caries is a disease occurring intermittently, in which host, microorganisms and substrate are all involved. Since saliva has the ability to affect all of them in several different ways, it becomes easy to understand the difficulties encountered in trying to evaluate any single anti-caries factor at any one time. Nevertheless, there is sufficient evidence to demonstrate a negative correlation between buffering capacity of stimulated and unstimulated whole saliva and caries. In addition, there is no doubt that when saliva is absent, or drastically reduced in quantity, caries can be rampant. Hence caries preventive measures must be taken when there is any interference in salivary function which diminishes flow and when buffering capacity is low.

5.4.2. Radiation Caries

Following radiotherapy for tumours in the vicinity of the salivary glands conditions conducive to a rapid onset of caries are created not only by the shortage of saliva but also by the resultant dietary change. Liquids and soft foods high in carbohydrate content are often consumed at frequent intervals throughout the day. This in turn leads to an alteration in the oral flora in favour of cariogenic *S. mutans* and lactobaccilli as well as candida which can exacerbate the mucositis caused by the irradiation.[7] If no special preventive regime is followed, rampant caries is very likely to develop.

It is now known that X-radiation in the doses administered in cancer therapy does not physically alter enamel to increase its caries susceptibility. Indeed, one laboratory study showed that irradiated enamel was more resistant than non-irradiated enamel to an artificial caries attack. However, the effect of X-radiation on dentine has not yet been tested. Nevertheless, it is most likely that the altered environment of the teeth, created as a result of salivary gland impairment, is responsible for the onset of rampant caries.

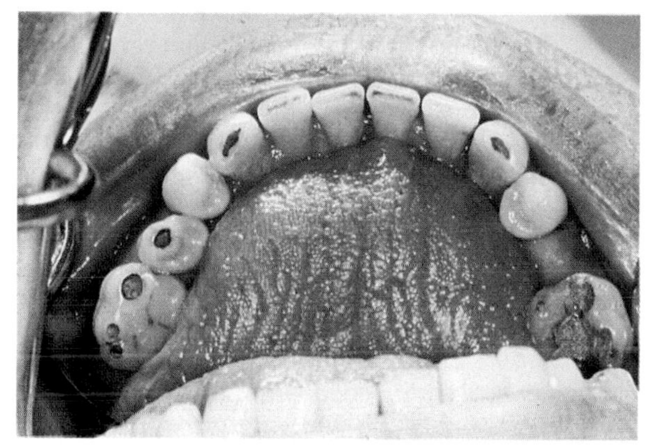

Fig. 5.1. A typical pattern of carious attack in a patient with xerostomia, in this case caused by radiotherapy in the region of the salivary glands. The cusp tips and incisal edges are typically attacked because dentine is often exposed by tooth wear in these areas. Dentine is more susceptible to caries than enamel.

The typical pattern of caries development is shown in *Figs.* 1.9 and 5.1. The cervical margins of the teeth are very rapidly attacked. The incisal edges of anterior teeth and the cusp tips of posterior teeth, which are normally very resistant to caries attack, also suffer rapid destruction. All these areas are covered by only a thin layer of enamel so that, without the protection of saliva, caries rapidly invades dentine. If any root surfaces are exposed they are even more rapidly attacked and are very difficult to treat (*see* Chapters 3 and 10).

5.4.3. Preventive Measures

There are three fundamental steps that have to be taken before putting into practice any preventive measures. The dentist must first recognize that a patient is 'at risk' (*see* Chapter 4.4), he must explain the situation to the patient and then encourage adoption of the following necessary preventive measures:

Dietary Control

It is important that dietary advice (*see* Chapter 6.5) be given. However, rigid dietary control may not be practical in irradiated patients although they can be advised to restrict the consumption of refined carbohydrate to mealtimes.

Chemical Plaque Control

In individuals with very dry mouths, normal oral hygiene practices becomes painful and consequently inadequate. In these extreme cases, chemical plaque control with a mouthwash containing chlorhexidine gluconate is invaluable since it inhibits the deposition of plaque. In addition *S. mutans* is very sensitive to chlorhexidine. Ideally, when the problem can be anticipated, patients about to have radiotherapy in the region of the salivary glands should be made dentally fit and begin to use the chlorhexidine mouthwash (10 ml at a concentration of 0·2 per cent) twice daily for about a week before radiotherapy. During radiotherapy, depending on the severity of the mucositis, the concentration can be reduced, so that the solution does not sting the mouth. Chlorhexidine is also effective against candida which also flourishes in dry mouths and may exacerbate radiation mucositis.

Streptococcus mutans counts, stimulated salivary flow rate and buffer capacity (*see* Chapter 4.4) should ideally be measured before radiotherapy so that baselines can be established. Measurements should then be repeated every month until the stimulated salivary flow rate reaches 0·7 ml/min. If the *S. mutans* count exceeds $2{\cdot}5 \times 10^5$/ml of saliva this should be reduced by self-application of a 1 per cent chlorhexidine gel in flexible vacuum moulded application trays (*Fig.* 5.2) specially made for each patient. The teeth should be exposed to the gel for 5 minutes daily for 14 days (*see* Chapter 9.4.5). Such treatment has been shown to keep the *S. mutans* count in control for at least three months in subjects with normal salivary flow. However, when salivary flow is diminished the chlorhexidine gel may have to be applied at intervals of less than three months.

The Use of Fluoride

The use of fluoride to aid remineralization and arrest early carious lesions is extremely valuable. Several studies have shown that, even if diet is uncontrolled, it is possible to prevent radiation caries by daily 5 minute self-application of a 1 per cent sodium fluoride gel (0·4 per cent F^-) in custom-made applicators (*see Fig.* 5.2). However, there must be total commitment to such a regime for several months until the flow of saliva returns. This may not be practical. Moreover, the same studies showed that if subjects did not comply completely with this regime, then caries was uncontrolled. It is therefore more practical to recommend daily sodium fluoride mouthwashes

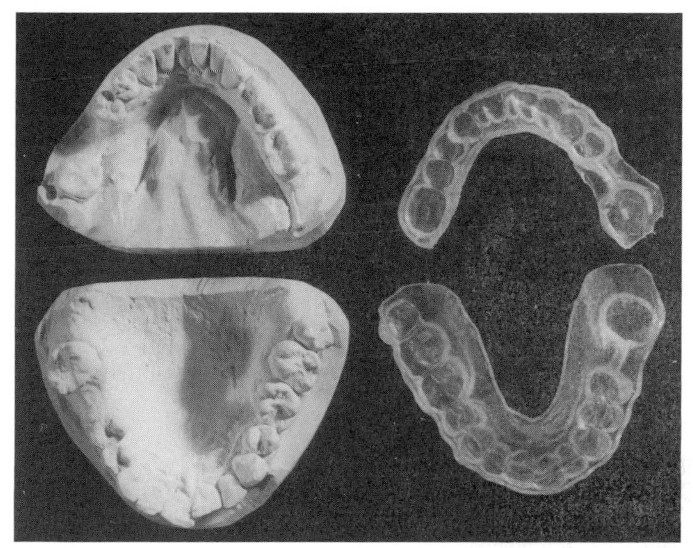

Fig. 5.2. Custom-made flexible vacuum-moulded trays for self-application of chlorhexidine or fluoride gel.

(0·05 per cent NaF) in the long term together with topical application of a fluoride gel (1·23 per cent F) by the dentist every three months.

When the shortage of saliva is not severe, dietary control and fluoride supplementation may be the only measures required. In extreme cases, chlorhexidine is also necessary. Without constant vigilance and regular monitoring by the dentist, a short lapse by the patient may have disastrous results.

REFERENCES

1. Thylstrup A. and Fejerskov O. (1986) *Textbook of Cariology.* Copenhagen, Munksgaard, Chapter 3.
2. Speirs R. (1984) Saliva and dental health (1). *Dent. Update* **11,** 541–552.
3. Speirs R. (1984) Saliva and dental health (2). *Dent. Update* **11,** 605–612
4. Shannon I. L., McCrary B. R. and Starcke E. N. (1977) A saliva substitute for use by xerostomic patients undergoing radiotherapy to the head and neck. *Oral Surg.* **44,** 656–661.
5. S'Gravenmade E. J. and Panders A. K. (1981) Clinical applications of saliva substitutes. *Front. Oral Physiol.* **3,** 154–161.
6. Marks N. J. and Roberts B. J. (1983) A proposed new method for the treatment of dry mouth. *Ann. R. Coll. Surg. Engl.* **65,** 191–193.
7. Brown L. R., Dreizen S., Handler S. et al. (1975) Effect of radiation-induced xerostomia on human oral microflora. *J. Dent. Res.* **54,** 740–750.

CHAPTER 6

DIET AND CARIES

6.1. ACID PRODUCTION IN DENTAL PLAQUE

Fermentable carbohydrate and a cariogenic plaque need to be present on a tooth surface for acid to form. The acid is produced by bacterial metabolism of the carbohydrate substrate. The process is well illustrated by the 'Stephan curve' shown in *Fig.* 1.2. A 10 per cent glucose rinse produces a rapid drop in the plaque pH to a level below which enamel will dissolve. Most importantly, the pH remains low for some 30–60 minutes before rising again to a safe level. Thus a single rinse, lasting a matter of seconds, can cause demineralization lasting over 30 minutes. Many foods and drinks containing sugar can produce this rapid drop in pH, which then remains low for some time. Indeed, other workers using electrodes placed interdentally have shown that the pH may remain depressed for some hours.

There has been a vast amount of experimental work linking fermentable carbohydrate and dental caries.[1, 2, 3] This work has not only proved conclusively that sugar is the most important dietary item in caries aetiology but also it has shown how patients may best be advised in the prevention of the disease by dietary control.

6.2. SOME EVIDENCE LINKING DIET AND CARIES

The evidence linking diet and dental caries has been taken from epidemiological studies, human clinical studies, animal experiments, and plaque pH studies.

6.2.1. Epidemiological Evidence

The consumption of sugar in substantial amounts is a recent trend in many areas of the world. Evidence linking sugar and caries has come from communities whose caries status has been recorded before and after an increase in the availability of sugar. One of the best known examples of this is the dental status of the inhabitants of Tristan da Cunha, a remote rocky island in the South Atlantic. Their dental state was excellent in the 1930s when their diet comprised potatoes and other vegetables, meat and fish. However, since 1940, there has been a sharp increase in the consumption of imported sugary foods and a commensurate increase in caries.

The severe dietary restrictions in many countries during World War II were accompanied by a decrease in dental caries. The teeth which had already erupted showed the same reduced caries score as the teeth developing at that time. The improvement was therefore due to a local dietary effect rather than a systemic nutritional one.

Epidemiological studies on other groups of people eating low amounts of sugar have also yielded interesting results. In 1942 an eccentric, wealthy Australian businessman transformed a spacious country mansion, called Hopewood House, into a home for young children of low socioeconomic background. When the children were 12 years old they could move to other accommodation but remain associated with the House. Since this entrepreneur attributed his own improvement in health to a drastic change in dietary habits, he stipulated that the children should be raised on a natural diet excluding refined carbohydrates. The dental surveys revealed a very low prevalence and incidence of dental caries, much lower than in children of the same age and socioeconomic background attending ordinary state schools in New South Wales. However, after 12 years of age, when close supervision ended, their caries rate became virtually the same as that in the children in the state schools. This indicates that the diet eaten up to the age of 12 years did not confer any subsequent protection.

Another piece of evidence linking diet and caries concerns the rare hereditary disease, fructose intolerance, which is caused by an inborn error of metabolism. Patients with this disease lack a certain liver enzyme and ingestion of foods containing fructose or sucrose causes severe nausea.

Consequently they avoid these foods. The caries experience of these patients is very low, indicating that a group of people who are not able to tolerate many sugary foods are unlikely to develop much caries.

6.2.2. Human Clinical Studies

Perhaps the most famous of all human clinical studies was begun in 1939 when the Swedish government requested an investigation into 'What measures should be taken to reduce the frequency of the most common dental disease in Sweden?' This led to a study on the relationship between diet and dental caries which was carried out at the Vipeholm Hospital, an institution for mentally defective individuals. The hospital, with its large number of permanent patients, provided an opportunity for a longitudinal study under well controlled conditions. A comparable study on human subjects will probably never be repeated as it would now be regarded as unethical to alter diets experimentally in directions likely to increase caries.

The patients were divided into one control and six experimental groups. Four meals were eaten daily and for one year patients received a diet relatively low in sugar with no sugar between meals. During this time the number of new carious lesions was assessed and found to be very low. Subsequently, the effect on caries of dietary changes involving the addition of large sucrose supplements in sticky or non-sticky form, either with or between meals, was assessed.

The control group, who continued with the basic diet, showed little increase in caries throughout the study. In the experimental groups the diet was supplemented by sucrose drinks or sucrose in bread or chocolate or caramels or 8 toffees or 24 toffees per day. There was a marked increase in caries in all groups except when the sucrose drink was taken at mealtimes. The risk of sugar increasing the caries activity was greatest if the sugar was taken between meals in a sticky form. Indeed, in the 24-toffee group, when the toffees were eaten between meals, the increase in caries was so great that the sugar supplement was withdrawn. This resulted in a fall in caries increment.

Dentists now base much of their dietary advice on the results of this study, stressing that the *frequency* of sugar intake should be reduced to confine sugar to mealtimes as far as possible. They advise against sticky, sweet foods and maintain that the rate of development of new disease will fall if this dietary advice is followed.

Another large-scale and important experiment on caries in humans was carried out in Turku, Finland, the aim being to compare the cariogenicity of sucrose, fructose and xylitol. Xylitol is a sugar alcohol which is sweet but is not metabolized to acid by plaque microorganisms. The results of the study showed that both sucrose and fructose were cariogenic but the almost total substitution of sucrose with xylitol resulted in a substantial reduction in caries incidence. This introduces the concept that it may be possible to substitute sucrose by substances which will impart sweetness but are not cariogenic. This is covered in more detail in section 6.5.2.

6.2.3. Animal Experiments

The most commonly used animal in caries experiments is the rat, but hamsters, mice and monkeys have been used also. One of the most important animal experiments was reported in 1954, when a system for rearing rats under germ-free conditions was reported. When these rats, who had no bacteria in their mouths, were fed a cariogenic diet, caries did not develop. This showed that a cariogenic oral microflora is essential for the development of the disease.

Subsequently, the importance of the local effect of diet in the mouth was demonstrated when animals fed a cariogenic diet via a stomach tube did not develop the disease. Rat experiments have also confirmed the positive correlation between frequency of sugar intake and caries severity.

Animal experiments are commonly used to compare the cariogenicity of foods. Such work has shown that sucrose, glucose, fructose, galactose, lactose and maltose are all cariogenic in varying degrees, with sucrose being the most cariogenic.

Animal experiments on the cariogenicity of starch have yielded conflicting results showing starch products with a cariogenicity ranging from very low to comparable to that of glucose! Heating at temperatures used in cooking and baking causes a partial degradation of starch so it is possible that cooked starch may be capable of fermentation to acid in the mouth and this has been confirmed by plaque pH studies (*see* section 6.2.4).

Recent experiments on rats have produced some interesting results when the animals were fed potato crisps. In the rat, which eats very frequently, some types of flavoured crisps cause caries. Crisps have long been regarded by dentists as a 'safe' snack and they are certainly less harmful than sweets. The eating pattern of man does not mimic the frequency of intake of the rat, so the results of this experiment should obviously be interpreted carefully. However, crisps should probably not be recommended as a safe snack, mainly because their high salt and fat content may be detrimental to the cardiovascular system.

6.2.4. Plaque pH Studies

The measurement of plaque pH before, during and after food is eaten should be a guide to the cariogenic potential of a food. Plaque pH can be measured intraorally by indwelling electrodes or extraorally on plaque samples. In these experiments 'Stephan curves' (*see* Chapter 1.2.2) can be produced by plotting plaque pH against time. Snack foods and drinks have been ranked according to the value of the minimum pH reached by the plaque. This means that information is now available to enable dentists to advise patients which snacks are likely to be cariogenic, which may be harmless and which may be positively beneficial.

Some snacks, like 'sugarless' chewing gum, appear not to depress plaque pH; others, like boiled sweets, sugared tea and coffee, and other sugared drinks clearly depress the pH. On the other hand some snacks, notably cheese and peanuts, actually tend to raise plaque pH, particularly if they are consumed after an acidogenic snack.

Plaque pH studies have also been used to differentiate between the potential cariogenicity of different sugars. Sucrose, glucose, fructose and maltose appear to be of similar acidogenicity, while lactose and galactose produce less severe pH falls. Cow's milk (containing lactose) and milk in unsugared tea cause slight plaque pH falls, but cow's milk has only a very weak cariogenic potential.

Starch products, especially those containing heat degraded starch, have also been shown to have an acidogenic potential. Thus starch snacks cannot be considered to be completely safe for teeth.

6.3. CULTURAL AND SOCIAL PRESSURES

Despite the fact that the misuse of sugar is known to be harmful, and has a possible role in obesity as well as dental caries, it still forms a considerable part of the diet of the people of the United Kingdom. Every man, woman and child eats an average of 900 g (2 lb) per week. One hundred grams (4 oz) of this is eaten in the form of confectionery and children consume on average 200 g (8 oz) per week. Some children eat as much as 200 g (8 oz) per day. Vast capital sums are invested in the sugar industry and related industries manufacturing soft drinks and confectionery. Large sums of money are also spent advertising sugar products, and the public are constantly exhorted to purchase sweet food products which they are told provide instant energy. Sweets are placed next to check-outs in supermarkets, and school tuck shops and chocolate bearing grannies flourish. In addition, many foods which are not generally thought of as cariogenic contain significant amounts of sucrose (sometimes called 'hidden sugar'), e.g. tomato soup, mustard, tomato sauce, frozen peas, tinned pasta, breakfast cereals, fruit yoghurts, many savoury baby foods and rusks.

6.4. DIET ANALYSIS

The practical problems of diet analysis and advice in the caries-prone patient should be tackled systematically. Initially, the patient's current diet should be determined because if sensible advice is to be given this baseline information is needed. Dietary analysis should be carried out on all patients with a high caries activity and in those with an unusual caries pattern.

There are two principal techniques for determining food intake. One is to record the dietary intake during the preceding 24 hours, the so-called

24-hour recall system. This involves careful history taking and relies on the patient's memory and honesty. The other method is to obtain a 3–7 day written diet record, the patient recording food and liquid intake as it is consumed. This relies on the patient's full cooperation as well as his or her honesty.

Both forms of diet recording suffer from the disadvantage that a 1–7 day record may not be representative of the diet consumed over a much longer time, although it is this which is likely to have been responsible for the caries and restoration status with which the patient presents. Thus, a diet history is an unscientific tool and must be interpreted with caution.

6.4.1. Recording the Diet

The authors use a diet sheet as shown in *Fig.* 6.1. When this is given to patients it is explained that their help is needed to find the cause of their dental decay. The cause is related to what they eat and drink and for this reason it is necessary for them to record everything eaten and drunk over a 4-day period, together with the time of eating. In addition, any medication should be entered. They are requested to keep the diet sheet with them and fill it in at the time to avoid missing anything. Quantities of food consumed are not specifically requested.

Notice that the patient is not told that the dentist is particularly interested in sugar intake as it would be human nature for the patient to eat less sugar in order to 'please'. The diet sheet has been designed to highlight the in-between-meal snack but the reason for this design is not explained to the patient at this stage. Two weekdays and the weekend are included because eating habits often vary when people are not at work or at school.

When the diet sheet is returned, it should not be discussed with the patient at that visit. It is not easy to come to grips immediately with the relevance of the eating pattern and to formulate advice on the spur of the moment. Consequently, it is good practice to study the sheet before the next visit so that it may be discussed in detail with the patient at that time.

6.4.2. Analysis of the Dietary Record

Initially all items on the diet sheet that contain sugar should be underlined in red. It is then possible to work out how many separate sugar intakes there are each day. This number should be recorded as it will be used to explain the importance of *frequency* of sugar intake to the patient before specific recommendations are made. Some dentists ask the patient to underline the items containing sugar. This can be good practice as it indicates whether the patient knows where hidden sucrose is to be found.

Special note is taken of the following:

a. The main meals, to see whether they are sufficiently substantial. This is important to prevent the patient craving food in between meals.

b. The between-meal snacks—are they cariogenic?

Diet Analysis *(See notes on other side)*

	THURSDAY		FRIDAY		SATURDAY		SUNDAY	
	Time	*Item*	*Time*	*Item*	*Time*	*Item*	*Time*	*Item*
BEFORE BREAKFAST								
Breakfast								
MORNING								
Mid-day Meal								
AFTERNOON								
Evening Meal								
EVENING & NIGHT								

Fig. 6.1. A form on which a patient may record diet over a 4-day period. This has been designed to highlight the between-meal snack, thus facilitating patient education when the sheet is completed and returned. On the reverse side of the diet sheet there are simple instructions explaining how it should be filled in.

c. Any medication, particularly if it is based on a sucrose syrup or if it is likely to cause dry mouth or thirst.
d. The number and type of between-meal drinks. Are these cariogenic?
e. The consistency of any between-meal snacks. Are they sticky and therefore take a long time to clear from the mouth?
f. The use of sucrose-containing chewing gum or any sweet that takes a long time to dissolve in the mouth.
g. Any sugary pre-bed snacks or drinks.

6.4.3. Dietary Recommendations

On the basis of the diet analysis, the clinician may be in a position to indicate to the patient the constituents of the diet which may be harmful and to make some positive recommendations. *Figs.* 6.2 and 6.3 show examples of two diet analysis sheets.

The diet sheet in *Fig.* 6.2 is from a middle-aged secretary with a high incidence of caries. This patient returned to the surgery after having kept the record, saying that *she* now realized the cause of the decay in her mouth. In addition she said how surprised she was to see how little she ate at mealtimes.

Fig. 6.3 shows one day in a remarkable diet in which the patient drank regularly every 2 hours day and night. The relevant feature of this diet sheet was that the patient was taking chlorpromazine (Largactil), an anti-psychotic drug, and lithium carbonate for depression. These drugs cause dry mouth and thirst respectively (*see* Chapter 5); the patient was consequently continually drinking and many of these drinks were cariogenic. Unfortunately the remains of the dentition were beyond repair and the patient is now edentulous.

Dietary recommendations should be recorded in the patient's notes together with the advice given.

6.5. DIETARY ADVICE

Dietary advice should be tailored to the needs of the individual patient and should form part of a comprehensive preventive programme consisting of oral hygiene instruction, the use of topical fluoride preparations and fissure sealants.

6.5.1. General Advice

Dietary advice must be practical, setting realistic goals. It is impossible to expect patients to cut out sugar from the diet completely, but it is feasible to reduce the total amount of sugar consumed, and to restrict sugar intake mainly to mealtimes.

Sugary foods or drinks between meals are particularly harmful and should be avoided in the caries-prone patient. Crisps, peanuts or cheese may be an acceptable alternative, although peanuts should not be given to

DIET ANALYSIS (See notes on other side) * = 2 spoons of sugar.

	THURSDAY		FRIDAY		SATURDAY		SUNDAY	
	Time	Item	Time	Item	Time	Item	Time	Item
BEFORE BREAKFAST	7·45	Tea *	7·00	Tea *	7·00	Tea *		
Breakfast	9·00	Coffee *	8·45	Coffee *	10·00	Tea * 2 pieces of toast		
MORNING	10·00 10·45	Coffee * Roll and butter Coffee *	9·30 10·45 11·45	Coffee * Roll and butter Coffee * Coffee *	11·00 12·00	Coffee * Coffee *	10·45 11·30	Tea * Tea *
Mid-day Meal	12·30 1·30	Coffee * Coffee *	1·45	Cheese & onion sandwich ½ Lager	1·0	Coffee * 1 muesli biscuit	2·0	Beef: roast potatoes Carrots: greens fresh pear Tea *
AFTERNOON	2·30 3·45 4·15	Coffee * Coffee * Coffee *	2·30 3·15 4·00 5·00	Coffee * Coffee * Coffee * Coffee *	3·00 4·15	Tea * Tea *	3·30	Tea *
Evening Meal	7·30	Country hash Tea *	9·00	Lasagne Tea *	7·00	Spare Ribs, Rice Tea *	5·00 6·30	Tea * Coffee *
EVENING & NIGHT	9·00 10·30	2 Muesli biscuits Tea * Pear	10·00 11·15	Tea * Tea * 2 biscuits	9·30 11·00	Tea * Tea *	8·00 10·00	Coffee * Cheese & biscuit Tea *

Fig. 6.2. A diet sheet completed by a middle-aged secretary with a very high incidence of caries. This lady returned to the surgery saying that she now realized that drinking frequent cups of sweetened tea and coffee was the likely cause of her caries.

	THURSDAY	
	Time	*Item*
BEFORE BREAKFAST	6.50 7.12. 7.30	Lucozade. Grapefruit juice Lucozade.
Breakfast	9.30	Cereal, milk, glucose, toast, marmelade; Coffee with glucose
MORNING	10.15 11.05 12.20 1.00	Tablets Lithium Valium Lemon drink Guiness Tablets Lithium
Mid-day Meal	1.45	Macaroni Cheese Tomato Shortbread Biscuits Water.
AFTERNOON	2.40 3.40 4.35	Lemon drink, Sugar & lemon juice Water Tea and glucose Lemon drink.
Evening Meal	6.45	Omelete, potato Biscuits, raisins, Water.
EVENING & NIGHT	8.10 8.45 9.45 9.55 10.05 1.10 3.30 5.30	Water Lime juice Peanuts: water Glacé cherry Tablets Lithium Valium Largactil Lucozade Lucozade Lucozade

Fig. 6.3. One day from an unusual diet sheet kept by a patient who was thirsty because of her medication and consequently drank regularly. Unfortunately most of the drinks were cariogenic.

children under five years as there is a real risk of death due to asphyxiation following inhalation of a single nut. Cutting out the bedtime snack or drink is particularly important since salivary flow is virtually absent at night and plaque pH may remain low for many hours.

It is neither necessary nor practical to stop children eating sweets altogether. However, it is not unreasonable to suggest that they are restricted to one day a week. In any case, children should be encouraged to eat a balanced meal before any sweets are given. If sweets are eaten, they will do least damage as part of a main meal. Grannie's advice of 'Don't eat them all at once' as she hands over the chocolates could be disastrous for dental health.

Adults should also be advised not to eat sugary snacks between meals, but it is often sweetened tea or coffee that is the problem in this group and here sugar substitutes can be very helpful.

6.5.2. Sugar Substitutes[3]

There is increasing interest in the use of sweetening agents which confer sweetness but do not produce acid when fermented by bacterial plaque. These products may be divided into two categories: those which have a calorific value (nutritive sweeteners) and those which do not (non-nutritive sweeteners).

Nutritive Sweeteners

The nutritive sweeteners include the sugar alcohols, and the most useful at present are sorbitol, mannitol and xylitol.

Sorbitol is a naturally occurring sugar alcohol found in some ripe fruits but produced commercially from sucrose or starch. It is about half as sweet as sucrose. It is slowly and incompletely absorbed from the gut and has been widely used as a sucrose substitute in diabetic preparations. The calorific value of food containing sorbitol is as high as that of sugar and thus it is not helpful for slimmers. There seems to be some uncertainty as to whether it is absolutely safe for teeth. Plaque bacteria cannot initially covert it to acid but there may be a possibility that they can adapt and start using it. However, it is regarded as much less cariogenic than sucrose. Drinks and chewing gums containing sorbitol are likely to be safer for teeth than their sucrose-containing counterparts.

Mannitol is another naturally occurring sugar alcohol that is thought to be relatively safe for teeth. Along with sorbitol it is a minor constituent of some sugar-free chewing gums.

Xylitol is a sugar alcohol with the same sweetness as sucrose, also naturally occurring but produced commercially from the wood of birch trees. Its extraction is a complicated process and therefore it is expensive. However, extensive clinical testing indicates that it is extremely safe for teeth since it cannot be metabolized to acid by plaque bacteria. In addition it produces almost no impact on blood sugar levels, so it is useful for diabetics.

It is a good food preservative and it produces a temperature drop when dissolved in the mouth, which adds to the interest of confectionery. For these reasons it is used in chewing gums, fruit gums, peppermints and some chocolates, being particularly popular in Finland and Switzerland where much of the original research was carried out. Some workers have demonstrated the ability of xylitol to aid remineralization, presumably because it stimulates salivary flow.

Another class of sucrose substitutes worthy of mention are the hydrogenated lycasins made from starch. They produce only a moderate pH drop in plaque and are used in some confectionery.

Preventive dentistry advanced significantly in Switzerland in 1969 when the Swiss Office of Health stipulated that non-acidogenic confectionery could be classed and advertised as 'safe for teeth'. To make this claim the products are tested for their ability to depress plaque pH. Only those products which do not cause a pH drop below pH 5·7 under certain specified conditions are allowed to be advertised in this way.

Non-nutritive Sweeteners

These are sometimes called 'intense sweeteners' because they have a sweetness many times that of sucrose. These substances impart sweetness but furnish no calories and are absolutely safe for teeth. Until recently only saccharin, which has the disadvantage of a bitter after-taste, was available. Recently, acesulfame-K, which is chemically similar to saccharin, has also become available. Another new product is aspartame (tradenames Canderel and Nutra Sweet). This is a particularly interesting product containing two amino acids, and it is thought to be particularly safe since it undergoes normal protein metabolism. Its taste is regarded as closest to that of sucrose, with no bitterness.

Each of these products may be invaluable to patients with a high caries incidence where a frequent sweet drink, such as sugared tea or coffee, is identified as the culprit. While some patients are able to give up sugar, others need the sweet taste to enjoy the drink and may find one of these non-nutritive sweeteners an acceptable alternative. Unfortunately, none of them impart the 'body' given to tea or coffee by two heaped teaspoons of sugar, so that many patients find it very difficult to give up the sugar habit.

The non-nutritive sweeteners are also used to sweeten manufactured drinks such as lemonade and orange squash. Obviously these products are preferable to their sugar-containing counterparts from a dental point of view.

6.5.3. Protective Foods

The consumption of some foods after sugar, such as cheese and nuts, has been shown to raise plaque pH. Cheese is useful in this respect because it can be recommended as the last course of a meal or as a 'safe' snack.

6.5.4. 'Safe' Snacks

It is really remarkably difficult to draw up a list of snacks that are safe in all respects. Although cheese is safe for teeth its high saturated fat content may not please cardiologists. This group may be similarly concerned at the recommendation of plain crisps owing to their high salt content. Fruit is *less* cariogenic than sweets but contains natural sugar. Dried fruits, such as raisins and apricots, have a high sugar content and cannot be considered as 'safe' snacks. Many fruits are very acid (lemons, sour apples, oranges, grapefruit) and excessive use of such fruits or their juices may cause acid erosion of the dental tissues. However, used in moderation fruit is safer than sweets. Nuts are a safe snack for older children and adults.

Bread and unsweetened biscuits are relatively safe for teeth provided they are not spread with jam or honey. Some raw vegetables such as carrots and tomatoes are 'safe' but are not to everyone's taste.

6.5.5. Advice to Pregnant and Nursing Mothers

There is little evidence in modern societies that children suffer any dental abnormalities due to maternal malnutrition. Nor is there evidence to suggest there will be any significant benefit to the teeth of the infant when a pregnant woman is given additional minerals, vitamins or fluoride. There is no apparent relationship between nutritional deficiencies during tooth formation and caries.

Breast feeding is strongly recommended by paediatricians since there is strong evidence that the number of infections and allergic conditions such as eczema are reduced in children who are breast fed, probably because of the antibodies present in human milk.

From a cariogenic point of view it is widely believed that breast feeding is safer than bottle feeding. This may be because breast milk contains lactose which is significantly less cariogenic than sucrose. However, *very rare* cases of rampant caries have been described in infants breast feeding on true demand for up to two years or more. In this condition the infants suckle regularly through the day and the night, perhaps 60 times per 24 hour period for several years.

The practice of adding sugar or honey to baby foods should be discouraged since this may cause the development of a 'sweet tooth' and influence the selection of cariogenic foods in later life. The use of a sucrose vehicle for vitamin supplements is also unwise since these have been implicated in the aetiology of rampant caries in infants and young children. Above all, the child should never be given a dummy or bottle containing a sugar solution to be sucked at will nor should a bottle of sweet drink be suspended in the cot so that the young child can drink at will throughout the night without waking the parent.

6.5.6. Young Children

Parents should be encouraged to give their children foods which do not foster a 'sweet' tooth. Some people believe that if children are given a savoury diet they will be happy to eat meals containing such foodstuffs in preference to sweet-tasting foods. Friends and relatives should be encouraged to bring small toys, fruit or crisps as presents rather then sweets. Drinks at bedtime, other than water, should be strongly discouraged.

6.5.7. Chronically Sick Children

Many children with chronic medical disorders are placed at considerable risk when dental treatment procedures have to be carried out. Every care should be taken to prevent caries in such patients, although the syrupy vehicles often used to administer medicines make caries more likely. There is a need for strict dietary control as well as thorough oral hygiene, fluoride supplementation and fissure sealing of susceptible teeth.

6.5.8. Patients with Dry Mouths

This group is particularly at risk to dental caries as discussed in Chapter 5. Thirst or the need to lubricate the mouth often results in the consumption of frequent sweet drinks or the chewing and sucking of sweets. Mouth lubricants and/or 'safe' drinks and gums should be recommended.

6.5.9. Dietary Changes

Diet may remain constant over many years but the dentist should watch for changes in caries status. If a patient starts to develop new lesions, the dietary cause should be sought. Perhaps the patient has left home and started work with a radical change in diet. Alternatively, retirement, bereavement or illness may have resulted in changed dietary habits. Sometimes mints are substituted for cigarettes when giving up smoking and the mint habit may persist long after the craving for a cigarette has gone.

6.5.10. Monitoring the Effect of Dietary Advice

Food intake and dietary habits are very difficult to influence. To find out whether the patient has followed the suggested dietary recommendations, the dentist can simply ask the patient about any changes. However, it has been claimed[4] that it is much better to carry out a follow-up microbiological examination by doing salivary tests to count the number of *S. mutans* and lactobacilli (*see* Chapter 4). Such tests are now routine in Sweden, where these techniques have been pioneered and where it is claimed that giving dietary advice without following the result microbiologically is like weight-watching without scales! If the patient is following the advice, the counts should fall.

6.6. DIETARY MISCONCEPTIONS

A number of misconceptions exist about diet and dental caries and it may be appropriate to end this chapter by laying a few ghosts!

One serious misconception is that only refined carbohydrates (sucrose or white sugar) are harmful to teeth while other carbohydrates are not. Sucrose is certainly regarded as the 'arch-criminal' because it is the most abundant sugar—it is used by food manufacturers all over the world as a food ingredient and it is readily used by bacteria to form extracellular polysaccharides which make plaque thicker and stickier. However, other sugars, such as glucose, glucose syrup and fructose, are also bad for teeth although they may be somewhat less damaging than sucrose.

Health foods are very fashionable nowadays; it has been suggested that fibrous foods such as apples and carrots 'clean' teeth thus removing plaque and preventing caries. While fibrous foods are preferable to a sucrose snack, there is no evidence that they can 'clean' the teeth. Another popular health food is honey. This so-called 'natural' sugar is just as cariogenic as other sugars. Many brands of muesli contain both sugar and honey. In the same way, the naturally occurring sugar in fruit juices probably makes these products just as cariogenic as the squashes.

Finally, it is very common for patients who are asked to give up sugar in tea and coffee to reduce the *amount* of sugar (say 1 teaspoon instead of 2) rather than giving it up completely. Thus, the frequency of sugar intake and therefore the frequency of pH fall may not be altered. It is important to check that patients really understand the message, otherwise they may make a considerable effort to no avail.

REFERENCES

1. Murray J. J. (1983) *The Prevention of Dental Disease.* Oxford, Oxford University Press, Chapter 2.
2. Nikiforuk G. (1985) *Understanding Dental Caries, Vol. 1.* Basel, S. Karger, Chapters 7 and 8.
3. Thylstrup A. and Fejerskov O. (1986) *Textbook of Cariology.* Copenhagen, Munksgaard, Chapter 8.
4. Krasse B. (1984) Can microbial knowledge be applied in dental practice for the treatment and prevention of dental caries? *J. Can. Dent. Assoc.* **3,** 221–223.

CHAPTER 7

FLUORIDE SUPPLEMENTATION

7.1. INTRODUCTION

In 1901 an American dentist, Dr F. McKay, who had recently arrived in Colorado Springs from Pennsylvania, noticed that the teeth of many of his patients had a particular appearance which he called 'mottled enamel'. He described this enamel as 'characterized by minute white flecks, or yellow or brown spots or areas, scattered irregularly or streaked over the surface of a tooth, or it may be a condition where the entire tooth surface is of a dead paper-white, like the colour of a china dish'.[1] It was not until the 1930s that excessive fluoride in the drinking water ($>2{\cdot}0$ parts/10^6 F or 2mg F/litre) was shown to be responsible for this 'mottling' and the condition was related to a low prevalence of dental caries. This work was done in the USA[2] and Britain.[3] The term 'dental fluorosis' was coined and research was begun to study the possible benefits of fluoride.

In 1942 Dean and his co-workers[4] published the classical epidemiological studies carried out by the US Public Health Service on children, 12–14 years of age, living in 20 towns, relating caries experience and the fluoride content of the water supply. They showed that when the drinking water contained about 1 part/10^6 fluoride the teeth of the lifelong inhabitants of that area had a low caries prevalence but no signs of dental fluorosis. For example, children aged 12–14 years had 50 per cent less caries than those with no fluoride in the water. These observations led to the addition of fluoride to fluoride deficient water supplies in several controlled clinical studies throughout the world.[5] The optimum level of fluoride recommended in temperate climates was 1 part/10^6 while in tropical climates, where water consumption was greater, the level was reduced to 0·7 parts/10^6. The results of these studies showed conclusively that it was possible to reduce caries by supplying optimal levels of fluoride.

However, water fluoridation does not completely prevent caries. Furthermore, many communities do not have piped water and for geographical and political reasons it has not been possible to fluoridate all water supplies. Consequently, a great deal of research has been carried out to develop alternative methods of supplementing fluoride intake. The aim of this chapter is to discuss this supplementation of fluoride in dental practice in terms of efficacy and safety. It is outside the scope of this book to discuss the extensive epidemiological investigations, human clinical trials and animal laboratory studies that have been carried out in relation to fluoride and caries or to cover the physiology of fluoride. The reader is referred to a book on fluorides by Murray and Rugg-Gunn[5] for detailed information on these topics.

7.2. CRYSTALLINE STRUCTURE OF ENAMEL[6]

Enamel mineral is crystalline and has a lattice structure characteristic of hydroxyapatite, the smallest repeating unit of which can be expressed by the formula:

$$Ca_{10}(PO_4)_6(OH)_2$$

However, it is not a pure hydroxyapatite since it also has a non-apatite phase (amorphous calcium phosphate or carbonate) and additional ions or molecules are adsorbed onto the large surface area of the apatite crystals. It is important to understand that enamel is essentially a porous structure, allowing ions to diffuse into it. Indeed, the composition of its hydroxyapatite lattice can vary throughout, markedly affecting its structure. This can happen in several different ways:

a. The crystal lattice has the capacity to substitute other ionic species of appropriate size and charge. Thus, within the lattice calcium can be exchanged for radium, strontium, lead and hydrogen ions while phosphate can be exchanged for carbonate, and hydroxyl for fluoride.

b. Sodium, magnesium and carbonate can be substituted or adsorbed at the crystal surface.

c. There may be defects present in the internal lattice.

d. It is also possible for part of the lattice to be lost without the whole crystal disintegrating.

7.3. DEPOSITION OF FLUORIDE IN ENAMEL

There is a great deal of scope for affecting the fluoride concentration of enamel since it can be deposited in three stages in its development. Low concentrations, reflecting the low levels of fluoride in tissue fluids, are incorporated in the apatite crystals during their formation. After calcification is complete, but before eruption, more fluoride is taken up by the surface enamel which is in contact with the tissue fluids. Finally, after eruption and throughout life, the enamel continues to take up fluoride from its external environment. At this time, the uptake of fluoride will be influenced by the state of the enamel, i.e. whether it is sound or whether acid etching or caries have made it more porous by preferentially dissolving its interprismatic constituents. Any such increase in porosity facilitates the diffusion and uptake of fluoride by enamel. Enamel from newly erupted teeth also takes up more fluoride than mature enamel.

Fig. 7.1 shows the fluoride concentration in enamel (sampled at different depths from the surface) in teeth of persons with differing exposure to fluoride from the water supply. The fluoride content of intact surface enamel is much higher than the interior enamel but tends to be extremely variable. It varies between primary and permanent teeth, between different individuals living in the same area, between different teeth in the same individual and even between different surfaces of the same tooth. In carious enamel, white spot or brown spot lesions, fluoride levels are raised, whereas in areas worn by attrition the levels are low.

7.3.1. Reaction of Fluoride with Enamel

In order for fluoride to be retained by enamel it has to be deposited as fluorapatite, the fluoride ion replacing the hydroxyl ion in the unit cell. Fluoride acquired from the tissue fluids during development and post-eruptively from the saliva and drinking water is incorporated in this form. However, because of the low concentrations of fluoride in these media it takes a long time for appreciable amounts of fluorapatite to accumulate in

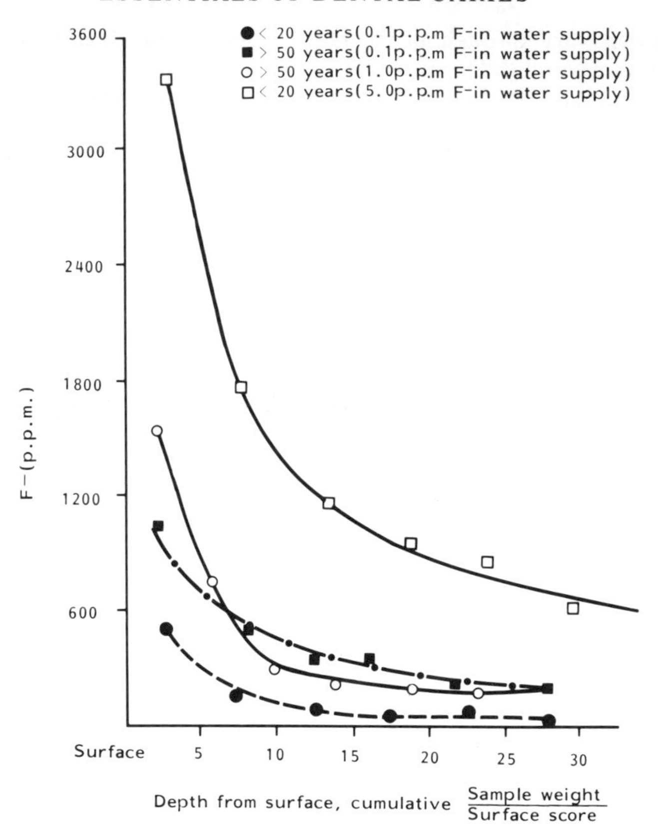

Fig. 7.1. Fluoride concentration in enamel (sampled at different depths from the surface) of teeth of persons with differing exposure to fluoride from the water supply. (From Isaac *et al.* 1958.[7])

enamel. Therefore, the aim of applying fluoride topically is to form significant amounts of fluorapatite within minutes. This is difficult to achieve because two different reactions are thought to take place between enamel and fluoride in solution depending on the fluoride concentration. On exposure to relatively *low concentrations of fluoride*, i.e. below 75 parts/10^6, hydroxyapatite is converted to fluorapatite:

$$Ca_{10}(PO_4)_6(OH)_2 + 2F^- \rightarrow Ca_{10}(PO_4)_6F_2 + 2OH^-$$

Larger amounts of fluoride are taken up from solutions containing *higher concentrations of fluoride* but only part of this fluoride is in the form of fluorapatite. Some fluoride ions are adsorbed onto the crystal surfaces but the rest combine with calcium ions from the lattice to form calcium fluoride

(CaF_2), liberating phosphate ions and partly disintegrating the lattice in the process:

$$Ca_{10}(PO_4)_6(OH)_2 + 20F^- \rightarrow 10CaF_2 + 6PO_4 + 2OH^-$$

Because it is slightly soluble, most of the CaF_2 dissolves and is lost within a few hours after a topical fluoride treatment but a certain amount of this fluoride does find its way into the enamel. It is also possible for fluorapatite crystals to be reprecipitated, given the right conditions. If, after treatment of the enamel with a fluoride solution, the enamel is sealed by painting with a varnish, more fluoride is retained by the enamel.

7.3.2. Acidulated-phosphate-fluoride (APF)

The uptake of fluoride by enamel is greatly increased when the pH is lowered. However, a low pH also results in demineralization of enamel with increased formation of calcium fluoride and the release of phosphate. In 1963 Brudevold and co-workers tried to suppress these damaging reactions by adding phosphate to the solutions. After laboratory tests on the effect on enamel of various concentrations of phosphate buffer, they concluded that 1·2 per cent fluoride as sodium fluoride in 0·1mol/l phosphate buffer, resulting in a solution of pH 3·2, fulfilled most of the requirements of a fluoride agent to be periodically applied to the tooth surface. Similar preparations with lower fluoride concentrations (0·01–0·3 per cent F) were also formulated for more frequent use as mouthrinses. All such 'acidulated-phosphate-fluoride' preparations are referred to as APF.

Over 50 per cent of the fluoride in an APF solution is present as undissociated hydrofluoric acid (HF) while most of the fluoride in a non-acidic sodium fluoride solution of equivalent fluoride concentration is present as F^-. Since HF diffuses into enamel more readily than F^-, fluoride from APF solutions penetrates more deeply into enamel than fluoride from a non-acidic sodium fluoride solution. Consequently, more fluoride is deposited in sub-surface as well as surface enamel.

7.3.3. Stannous Fluoride

In order to find a fluoride compound which was a more effective anti-caries agent than sodium fluoride, several fluoride salts were tested in the 1940s for their ability to reduce enamel solubility in the laboratory. Stannous, lead, ferric and zirconium fluorides were tested and it was thought that the relatively insoluble phosphate precipitates formed on the enamel by these cations would augment the caries protective action of fluoride. In fact, although these compounds were shown to be more effective in reducing enamel solubility in the laboratory, subsequent clinical studies showed that lead, ferric and zirconium fluorides were not as effective as sodium fluoride in reducing caries incidence. Only in the case of the acidic stannous fluoride was a claim for superiority made but it has since been demonstrated that it is *not* more effective than APF *in vivo*. It is still questionable whether there is a cationic effect or if the fluoride alone is the effective component in stannous fluoride.

7.4. CARIOSTATIC MECHANISMS OF FLUORIDE[8]

Several methods of supplementing enamel fluoride, using many different vehicles containing varying concentrations of fluoride, have been tested over four decades and there is no doubt that such additional fluoride exerts a protective action against dental caries. There is also sufficient evidence to show that fluoride acts in several different ways both before and after tooth eruption. However, since dental caries is caused by several factors it has been difficult to determine precisely which mechanism of action predominates. It may well depend on the particular stage of enamel dissolution, the type of fluoride agent used as well as its fluoride concentration and the frequency of use.

In addition, fluoride in the oral environment is present in many forms. Besides the fluoride present in the apatite and non-apatite phases of the enamel itself, fluoride is present in plaque (5–10 parts/10^6 F), saliva (0·02 parts/10^6 F) and gingival crevicular fluid (0·008 parts/10^6 F). Consequently, more than one mechanism of action may operate simultaneously.

7.4.1. Pre-eruptive Effects

If fluoride is present during tooth development, it results in the formation of enamel with improved crystallinity which may be more resistant to acid attack. Optimum levels of fluoride encourage the growth of larger, more perfect, crystallites with a lower carbonate content and consequently a reduced acid solubility. It has also been suggested that the presence of fluoride during tooth formation results in slightly smaller teeth with more rounded cusps and shallower fissures. Although animal studies support this view, the results of human studies have not been consistent. Discontinuation of water fluoridation has been shown to result in an increase in caries, suggesting that pre-eruptive effects of fluoride are small.

7.4.2. Post-eruptive Effects

Effect on Demineralization and Remineralization

For many years the rationale behind the application of fluoride topically to enamel was to increase its fluoride content and consequently decrease its solubility in acid. However, this explanation is now considered to be too simplistic. Several clinical studies report a lack of correlation between total fluoride uptake by surface enamel and decrease in caries incidence, and the results of recent laboratory studies suggest that there may be an optimum level of fluoride uptake beyond which no additional benefit can be conveyed. Moreover, since it is now known that dental caries is characterized by alternating periods of demineralization or destruction and remineralization or repair, views on the mode of action of fluoride have changed.

During the process of enamel demineralization, its dissolved constituents, together with the buffering ions diffusing into plaque from the saliva, neutralize the acids which have been produced by plaque microorganisms. Consequently, plaque becomes supersaturated with respect to apatite which means that mineral depostion can occur. Two actions of fluoride are important here. Its presence in acid helps to inhibit demineralization and it also promotes remineralization, thus encouraging repair or arrest of the initial lesion.

Effect on Plaque Bacteria and Bacterial Metabolism

Depending on its concentration and pH, fluoride can exert a bactericidal or antienzymatic effect. At the concentration (over 1 per cent F) used for topical applications in the dental clinic both APF (pH 3·2) and stannous fluoride (pH 2·1) have been shown to be toxic to *S. mutans* but this must be a transient effect. Low concentrations (2–10 parts/10^6) can inhibit the enzymes involved in acid production and the transport and storage of glucose and glucose analogues in oral streptococci. It can also interfere with the synthesis of intracellular polysaccharides and so restrict the build-up of a reserve supply for acid production. Thus the presence of low concentrations of ionic fluoride in plaque can reduce the effect of a cariogenic challenge by reducing acid production and the consequent fall in pH. In order to be effective, the fluoride has to be in ionic form. Athough much of the fluoride in plaque is a loosely bound fraction, it can be liberated when the pH is reduced to 4 or 5 and so augment the low concentration of ionic fluoride (0·08–0·8 parts/10^6 F) normally present in plaque fluid.

Effect on Plaque Deposition

The ability of powdered hydroxyapatite to adsorb salivary protein is significantly reduced when it is treated with fluoride. Consequently, it was suggested that fluoride may also have the ability to retard the adsorption of salivary proteins on the enamel surface and hence slow down the deposition of pellicle and plaque. However, the results of clinical studies are equivocal and there is no evidence that plaque deposits are different in amount in high and low fluoride areas.

7.5. WHICH FLUORIDE SUPPLEMENT?[9]

Before considering supplementing fluoride, it is relevant to take into account the natural sources of fluoride in food. Seafood and tea are the principal dietary sources of this ion. In fish, it is the skin and bones which contain significant amounts of fluoride. These parts of the fish become edible during canning so that canned fish may contain 9 parts/10^6 F. An average infusion of tea, depending on the brand, contains between 1·4–

4·3 parts/10^6 F. Although tea consumption in the UK is high, there is no evidence that this has a beneficial effect on the dental health of the population. This may be because sugar is frequently added to tea.

Fluoride in fish will only be relevant if fish forms a major part of the diet. Similarly only individuals consuming a very large volume of *unsweetened* tea might be expected to benefit dentally. Thus, for most people, dietary fluoride supplementation is not practical and some other form of fluoride supplement should be considered.

To obtain the maximum benefit from fluoride, its transient presence is required soon after the initial caries attack. Since there is no way of knowing exactly when this is occurring, the aim has to be regular and frequent exposure of the enamel to fluoride to arrest the early lesion. Indeed, there is clinical evidence to suggest that regular use of preparations containing low concentrations of fluoride is more effective than irregular use of agents containing higher concentrations. Furthermore, it has also been shown that when exposure to fluoride is discontinued, its caries-reducing effect gradually wanes.

These factors have to be taken into consideration when choosing a fluoride supplement and the regime to be employed. Ultimately, however, the choice must be governed by the dental needs of the individual patient. Since available vehicles for fluoride supplementation contain varying amounts of fluoride it is also necessary to consider the safety of the fluoride preparation chosen.

Table 7.1 Vehicles used to carry fluoride to its sites of action

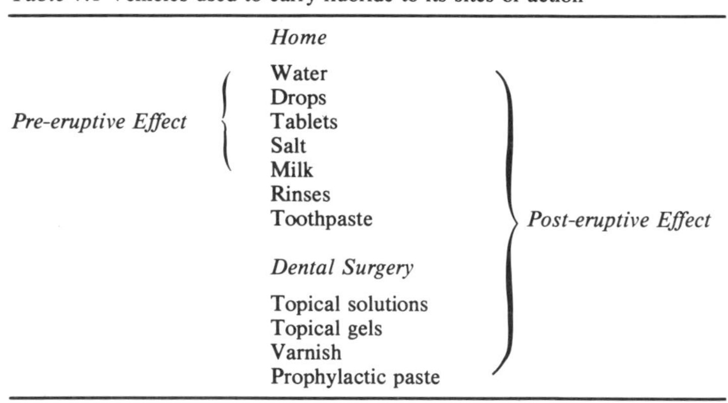

	Vehicle	
	Home	
Pre-eruptive Effect	Water	*Post-eruptive Effect*
Pre-eruptive Effect	Drops	*Post-eruptive Effect*
Pre-eruptive Effect	Tablets	*Post-eruptive Effect*
Pre-eruptive Effect	Salt	*Post-eruptive Effect*
Pre-eruptive Effect	Milk	*Post-eruptive Effect*
	Rinses	*Post-eruptive Effect*
	Toothpaste	*Post-eruptive Effect*
	Dental Surgery	
	Topical solutions	*Post-eruptive Effect*
	Topical gels	*Post-eruptive Effect*
	Varnish	*Post-eruptive Effect*
	Prophylactic paste	*Post-eruptive Effect*

Listed in *Table* 7.1. are the various vehicles used to carry fluoride to its sites of action. When fluoride is used at home in mouthrinses and toothpaste or applied in the dental surgery in the form of topical solutions, gels, varnishes or prophylactic pastes, its effect will only be post-eruptive unless some of these preparations are swallowed during tooth formation in the young. Fluoride will, in addition, have a pre-eruptive effect on developing enamel, if ingested in one of the following forms: fluoridated water, sodium fluoride tablets or drops, fluoridated salt or fluoridated milk.

Of all the above, fluoride in drinking water is the most effective, safest and cheapest way of reducing caries. Its effect is both pre-eruptive, if available during the period of tooth development, and post-eruptive and it has the added advantage that no conscious cooperation on the part of the individual is required. Indeed, it satisfies the criteria for the ideal fluoride supplement—a low, safe concentration used regularly and frequently to arrest the early lesion. However, since only 9 per cent of the population in the United Kingdom drinks fluoridated water, dentists are still faced with choosing alternative methods of supplementing the natural supply of fluoride.

7.6. FLUORIDE FOR INGESTION

7.6.1. Fluoride Tablets and Drops

A practical alternative to water fluoridation is the ingestion of fluoride in the form of sodium fluoride tablets or drops of a sodium fluoride solution, However, these forms of fluoride supplement should *never* be prescribed when the level of fluoride in the water *exceeds 0·7 parts/10⁶*. The Council on Dental Therapeutics of the American Dental Association recommends a daily intake of 0·25 mg F from 2 weeks up to the age of 2 years, 0·5 mg F from 2 to 3 years and 1 mg F from 3 to 16 years in areas where the level of fluoride in the water supply is less than 0·3 parts/10^6. However, the current recommended dosages in Sweden, Denmark, Norway, Finland and Switzerland are slightly lower.

There is no justification for exceeding the dosages recommended in the USA. Futhermore, in view of the increased use of fluoride toothpaste, some of which may be swallowed by small children, it is logical to delay increasing the dose in tablets to 1 mg until the age of 4 years by which time a child is more able to spit out and as a consequence swallows less paste. The dosage schedule recommended in the UK by Dowell and Joyston-Bechal[10] is shown in *Table* 7.2. For an infant the appropriate number of drops should be added to the liquid feed—fruit juice, milk or water. However, once teeth have erupted, the child should be encouraged to let a tablet dissolve slowly in the mouth, preferably at bedtime. This provides a topical effect on the enamel of erupted teeth followed, after swallowing, by a systemic effect on the developing teeth. A recent study in this country showed that the administration of 1 mg F tablets daily at school resulted in DMFS reductions of 81 per cent in the teeth erupting during the three-year trial.

Fluoride tablets should be prescribed until 12–16 years of age which means that, unlike water fluoridation, this regime requires the active and

Table 7.2 Recommended fluoride dosage schedule[10]

Age	*Concentration of fluoride in drinking water (parts/10⁶)* 0–0·3	0·3–0·7	0·7
2 weeks–2 years	0·25	0	0
2–4 years	0·50	0·25	0
4–16 years	1·00	0·50	0

Note: 2·2 mg sodium fluoride contains 1 mg F^-.

sustained cooperation of parent and child for this period. There is evidence to suggest that cariostatic benefits diminish after fluoride supplementation is stopped so, depending on the susceptibility of the individual to caries, provision may have to be made for some form of topical application of fluoride beyond the age of 16.

Some would advocate increasing the daily dose of fluoride for children who are medically at risk or handicapped, but there is little evidence to support this practice. A study carried out in the UK in a group of infants with cleft palate showed that it was possible to prevent caries almost totally by a programme which included fluoride tablets at a higher dose. This programme also included monthly parental dietary and oral hygiene counselling. In addition, there were 6-weekly, followed by monthly topical fluoride applications from the age of 2½ years to 3 years, as well as fissure sealing. Consequently, it is erroneous to attribute these subjects' resistance to caries solely to the particular dose of fluoride tablets used. However, it is interesting to note that a combination of fluoride regimes with dietary and oral hygiene counselling was so effective in preventing caries. On the other hand, one of the earliest studies of the relationship between caries experience and the fluoride content of water supplies showed quite clearly that near maximum reduction in caries experience occurred with a concentration of 1 part/10^6 F in the drinking water, with only little more benefit demonstrable at greater levels. It would seem therefore that the dentist should be more critical of the assumption that 'if a little fluoride is good, more fluoride is better.'

7.6.2. Fluoridated Salt

In Hungary and Switzerland fluoridated salt has been used for several years as an alternative to water fluoridation with some success. Careful studies have also been carried out in Columbia and Spain. The current concentration is 250 parts/10^6 F/kg but higher doses are being tested. Individual variation in intake is, however, a problem. Nevertheless, in parts of the world without piped water supplies, this may be a useful alternative to water fluoridation.

7.6.3. Fluoridated Milk

Milk, with a fluoride concentration of around 2·5 parts/10^6, has been used in some parts of Austria, West Germany, Japan and Switzerland. A recent clinical trial in Glasgow showed a 34 per cent reduction in caries in the first permanent molars of primary school children as a result of drinking 200 ml of milk containing 7 parts/10^6 F each school day for 4 years. However, there is great variation in the amount of milk consumed by children and considerable effort is required to ensure regular intake of the appropriate volume of fluoridated milk. Furthermore, not all children like milk, so some would be ingesting little or no fluoride from this source.

7.7. FLUORIDE PREPARATIONS FOR TOPICAL APPLICATION

7.7.1. Low Concentration Preparations for Frequent Use

Toothpaste

Most fluoride toothpastes currently on sale in the world contain fluoride as sodium monofluorophosphate (NaMFP) since it is compatible with the most commonly used abrasive systems. It has also been suggested that the MFP anion (PO_3F^{2-}) has anti-cariogenic properties of its own, exchanging with phosphate groups in the apatite crystals and resulting in a subsequent slower release of fluoride ion. In order to enhance the effect of MFP, some new toothpaste formulations also contain sodium fluoride and/or calcium glycerophosphate; there is some data suggesting the increased effectiveness of these mixtures.

Clinical trials of fluoride-containing dentifrices show a reduction in caries incidence ranging from an average of 17 per cent in subjects in optimum fluoride areas to about 34 per cent in non-fluoride areas. Consequently, the use of a fluoridated toothpaste should be recommended for all. However, its use should be supervised in pre-school children who are generally not capable of rinsing adequately and may swallow the paste. The majority of toothpastes currently available contain about 1 mg F/g (1 g is equivalent to about 12 mm of paste on the brush) although some products are available which contain 1·45 mg F/g. It has been estimated that, on average, a pre-school child may ingest 0·3–0·4 g of paste at each brushing resulting in a daily intake from toothpaste in excess of 0·5 mg F. At this level, although there is no danger to health, enamel fluorosis of the developing dentition is possible *if these children are also ingesting fluoride tablets* (*see* section 7.9.1 and *Fig.* 7.3*a–c*). It is impracticable to recommend a non-fluoride toothpaste for individual members of a family. Therefore, where fluoride tablets are used for the pre-school child, parents should be advised to limit the quantity of paste to approximately 0·3 g, which is the size of a small pea. The frequency of brushing with a fluoride paste should be limited to twice a day in these young children.

Mouthrinses

The daily, weekly or fortnightly use of a fluoride mouthrinse has proved to be one of the most valuable anti-caries measures in areas where the water supply has a low fluoride content, i.e. $<0{\cdot}1$ parts/10^6. The fluoride concentration advocated in the mouthrinse depends on its frequency of use. Individuals should be instructed to rinse for one minute with 10ml of a sodium fluoride solution at a concentration of 0·05 per cent sodium fluoride if used once daily or at 0·2 per cent if used at weekly or fortnightly intervals.

The results of clinical trials show that the cariostatic benefits of fluoride mouthrinses range between 16 and 50 per cent, depending on the length of the trial. Daily rinsing has been shown to be marginally more effective than weekly or fortnightly rinsing. Moreover, because of the lower concentration of fluoride, the daily mouthrinse is safer for children. For adults, choice should depend upon patient cooperation. APF preparations generally deposit more fluoride in enamel than neutral sodium fluoride solutions (*see* section 7.3.2). However, in clinical trials of fluoride rinses, they were found to be equally effective.

INDICATIONS

Fluoride mouthrinses are indicated in caries-prone children over the age of 6 years and caries-prone adults. Patients with orthodontic appliances would also benefit. It must be stressed that a dietary history should always be obtained. Suitable dietary advice as well as oral hygiene instruction should precede a prescription for fluoride.

CONTRAINDICATIONS

Mouthrinses are contraindicated in children (under 6 years of age) who are not capable of rinsing adequately They are also unnecessary when fluoride tablets are dissolved in the mouth.

7.7.2. High Concentration Preparations for Periodic Use: Sodium Fluoride, APF, Stannous Fluoride, Fluoride Varnish, Prophylactic Paste

Listed in *Table* 7.3 are the agents available, together with their respective fluoride concentrations and the approximate amounts of fluoride in each

Table 7.3 Agents available for topical fluoride application

Agents available	*Concentration*	*mg F^-/ml*
Sodium fluoride solution	2·0% NaF	10
Stannous fluoride solution	8·0% SnF_2	20
APF solution/gel	1·23% F	12
Sodium fluoride varnish	2·26% F	22
Prophylactic pastes	0·64–1·2% F	1

millilitre of the agent. This will be discussed later in relation to safety (*see* section 7.9.2). These preparations are supplied by the manufacturer in various forms: solutions of sodium fluoride, stannous fluoride and APF which are swabbed on the tooth surface; APF gels which can be swabbed on or applied in closely fitting trays; sodium fluoride varnishes which are applied with a brush; and prophylactic pastes containing fluoride which are applied with a rotating rubber cup. Apart from the prophylactic pastes, the other agents, when applied twice a year, have been shown to reduce dental caries by about 40 per cent.

In evaluating a topical fluoride treatment an important consideration is the length of time its caries-reducing effect is maintained and not merely the amount of fluoride deposited in enamel by such treatment. The drop-off in protection during the post-treatment period is less with APF than with the other fluoride agents. Consequently it has been the preferred topical agent during the last decade. It is available as a solution and gel and both have been found to be equally effective.

Stannous fluoride is now used less frequently because it presents several difficulties. It has an astringent taste and a tendency to stain because the stannous ion probably reacts with dietary sulphides. Furthermore, it is irritating to the gingival tissues and because it is readily hydrolysed it must be freshly prepared.

In order to minimize the loss of fluoride after topical application, fluoride varnishes have recently been developed. Duraphat, the product currently available in the UK, contains sodium fluoride in an alcoholic solution of natural varnishes. Clinical studies show that its effect is similar to that obtained with other topical fluoride preparations. However, it is particularly useful in treating children, whose cooperation is limited, because it can be applied quickly.

Prophylactic pastes are not recommended as agents to supplement fluoride since the use of any abrasive agent results in the loss of surface enamel which contains a high concentration of fluoride. Consequently the net loss of fluoride may be equal to, or greater than, the net gain. If a prophylactic paste is to be used, the choice should always be one which contains fluoride and is only mildly abrasive. Unless staining is severe, a fluoride toothpaste can effectively be used for prophylaxis.

Methods of Application

In the past a thorough prophylaxis was always advocated before topical fluoride application. However, it has been shown that fluoride ions diffuse easily through pellicle and plaque and that fluoride uptake by the underlying enamel is not affected by its presence. However, since plaque is responsible for caries and periodontal disease it is rational to let the patient remove any plaque present with a toothbrush before fluoride application. This approach would combine oral hygiene instruction with fluoride therapy.

SOLUTIONS

After cleaning, sodium fluoride, APF or stannous fluoride solutions are applied directly to the teeth, one quadrant being treated at a time. The teeth in each quadrant are isolated by cotton wool rolls and saliva is controlled by suction or a saliva ejector. After drying, the solution is applied with cotton pellets so that the teeth are continuously bathed in it for 4 minutes. In the case of stannous fluoride the recommended time is 2 minutes. Any excess should be aspirated to prevent the patient from swallowing it. Rinsing should be avoided.

GELS

Whereas the solutions are swabbed on a quadrant at a time, the gel can be applied to a complete arch in a closely fitting applicator tray. Consequently, fluoride gels are now used more extensively in practice than solutions. However, it has recently been shown[11] that even with well fitting custom-made trays, on average 78 per cent of the initial dose applied is ingested when no saliva ejector is used. As each millilitre of the gel contains 12 mg F, it is not advisable to advocate this form of fluoride application for children or for home use. In the surgery it is safer and more acceptable to children if the fluoride gel is applied with cotton pellets only on selected teeth which have been isolated and dried. In this way, the gel is easier and safer to apply than a solution because it adheres to the teeth and avoids the continuous wetting required when a solution is used.

If gel is used in applicator trays for adults (*see Fig.* 5.2), only a thin ribbon of gel should be placed in the tray and a saliva ejector or suction should always be used to prevent any gel from being swallowed. In addition, the teeth should be wiped with gauze to remove any excess gel after the tray is withdrawn.

VARNISH

Fluoride varnish is ideally applied on cleaned and dried teeth with a brush. However, the manufacturers of Duraphat claim that it is water tolerant and will cling onto teeth even if moisture is present. Consequently, it is easier and quicker to apply than the other fluoride agents. However, care should be taken in its application since it has a high fluoride content (22 mg per ml).

Indications and Contraindications

INDICATIONS

a. Caries-prone children (over 6 years), and caries-prone adults who cannot or will not use a fluoride mouthrinse, as well as patients with removable orthodontic appliances (biannual applications).

b. Children (over 6 years) and adults exposed to a greater cariogenic challenge because their dietary habits have changed since their last visit due to illness, change of school or occupation.

c. Patients suffering from salivary gland malfunction due to drugs, disease or radiotherapy (*see* Chapter 5) which results in diminished salivary flow.
d. Localized application to initial carious lesions which the clinician hopes to arrest.

A dietary history should be taken and advice given with oral hygiene instruction before fluoride application.

CONTRAINDICATIONS

The home use of these preparations, which contain relatively high concentrations of fluoride, is contraindicated for all patients for safety reasons. They are also contraindicated in the surgery for children under the age of 6 years who cannot spit effectively. Trays should not be used for the application of APF gels in children under the age of 16 years.

7.7.3. Topical Fluoride Application in Optimally Fluoridated Areas

Results of studies on the value of topically applied fluorides for children in such areas are not clear cut. Nevertheless, the highly susceptible individual should be given professsional applications of a topical fluoride preparation or asked to use a fluoride mouthrinse. It is important, however, to exclude children under the age of 6 years.

7.8. PRENATALLY ADMINISTERED FLUORIDE[12]

The benefit from pre-natal supplementation of fluoride is uncertain. It has been shown that some fluoride ingested by the pregnant woman passes through the placenta to the fetus. However, the concentration of fluoride in fetal tissues is low and does not seem to be linearly related to the fluoride intake by the mother. In the light of present knowledge, and the small benefit that could be gained, there is insufficient justification for the administration of fluoride tablets during pregnancy.

7.9. SAFETY

7.9.1. Enamel Fluorosis[13]

The first sign of an excessive intake of fluoride during the period of tooth formation is the eruption of teeth with fluorosed or mottled enamel. Although the precise mechanism by which enamel fluorosis occurs is not yet fully understood, it is believed that it affects the complex ameloblast function during enamel maturation leading, in some way, to defective mineralization. The permanent incisors and canines may be vulnerable until the age of 5–7 years.

Enamel fluorosis can be caused by a single high fluoride dose, multiple but lower doses and by low level continuous exposure. Consequently, it can be produced by fluoride in the drinking water (*see Fig.* 7.2) as well as by use

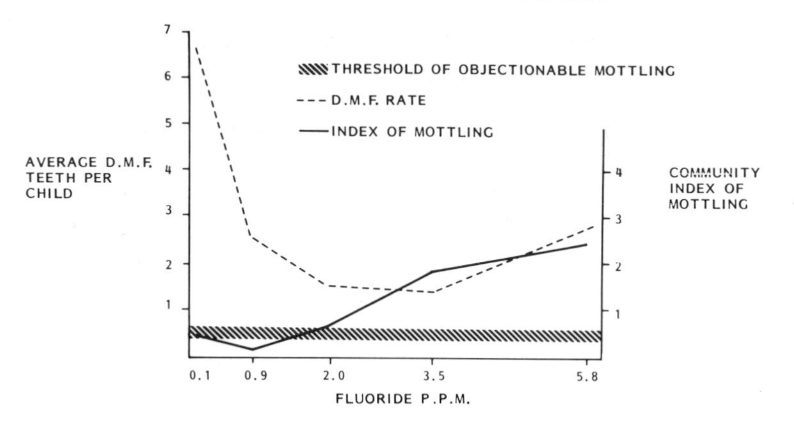

Fig. 7.2. Fluoride content of water: caries experience and enamel mottling in British children aged 12–14 years. (From Forest 1956.[16] Reproduced by courtesy of the Editor, *British Dental Journal.*)

of fluoride supplements. Since supplements are generally administered as single doses, either daily or periodically they produce much higher plasma peaks than the multiple divided doses received from the water supply.[14] Moreover, since fluoride from preparations for topical application[11] as well as from toothpaste[15] are readily absorbed, care must be taken in their use.

When fluorosis is mild, enamel merely loses its lustre and, when dried, opaque white flecks or patches can be seen (*Fig.* 7.3*a*). It is difficult to distinguish cases of mild fluorosis from other opacities of enamel due to infections in childhood, genetic causes or trauma.[17] However, such opacities are not usually aesthetically objectionable.

More obvious mottling or striations (*Fig.* 7.3*b*), with or without yellow or brown stains, are apparent in moderate cases of enamel fluorosis. When the condition is very severe, pitting occurs and the enamel is so hypoplastic that pieces break off very easily (*Fig.* 7.3*c*). The fluorosis illustrated in *Fig.* 7.3*a–c* was caused by excessive fluoride supplementation. The subjects all gave a history of supplemental fluoride drops or tablets at a daily dose of 0·5 mg F from birth to 2 years and 1 mg F thereafter which was the dosage originally recommended before the advent of fluoridated toothpaste. Since these children were also having their teeth brushed with a fluoridated paste twice a day from the age of 6–8 months, it is not difficult to see why fluorosis resulted, as their total daily intake would have been in excess of 1·0mg F (*see* page 93).

The cases illustrated in *Fig.* 7.3*a–c* suggest that there may be a variation in the response of these three children to fluoride. However, the histories revealed that there was a variation in their ability to rinse and spit out. The

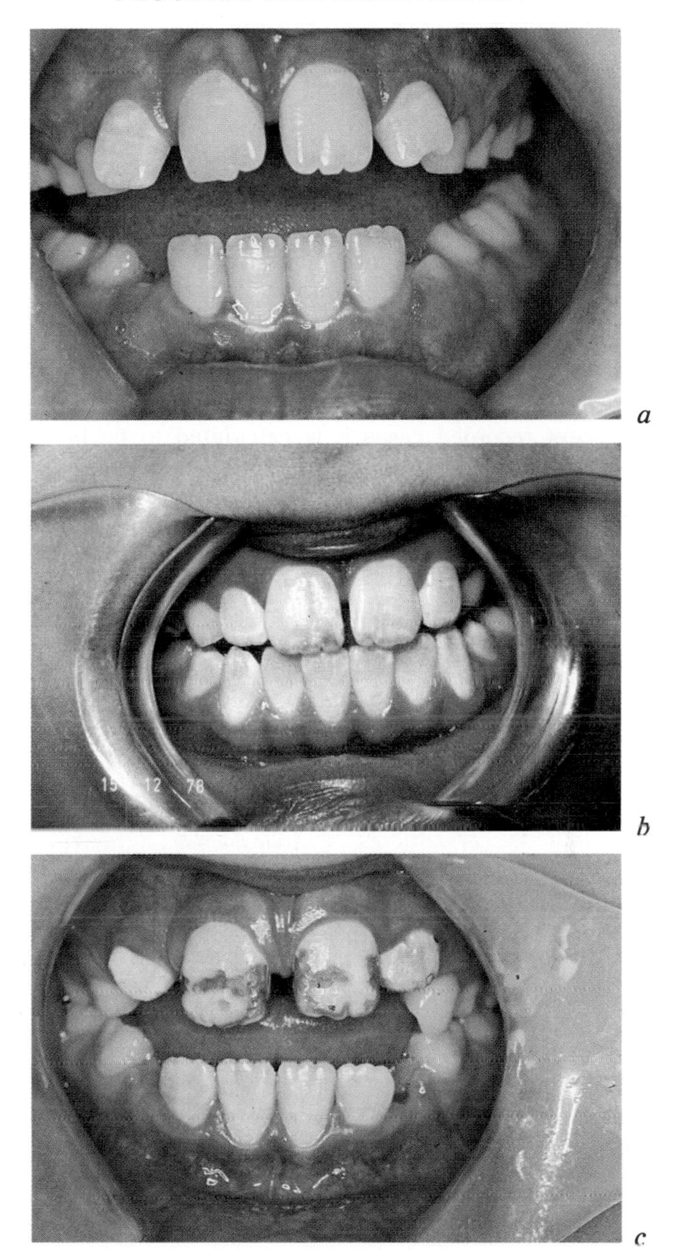

Fig. 7.3. *a.* Mild fluorosis. Note white flecks on upper anterior teeth. *b.* Moderate fluorosis. Note white striations and yellow-brown discolouration on 1|1. *c.* Severe fluorosis.

child with severe fluorosis (*Fig.* 7.3*c*) had difficulty rinsing until the age of 8 years. Therefore, in order to avoid fluorosis, it is necessary to restrict the quantity of fluoridated toothpaste used in children who are also ingesting a fluoride supplement.

7.9.2. Toxicity

Information on the toxicity of fluorides in humans is gathered from recorded cases of deliberate or accidental overdosage. On this basis the *acute lethal dose* of fluoride was calculated in 1965 by Hodge et al.[18] to be about 50 mg F/kg body weight. However, the National Poisons Information Service in this country is now more conservative and advises that the potentially lethal dose should be 14·28 mg F/kg to encourage the maximum caution in clinical work. The amount of fluoride which can produce early symptoms of *acute fluoride poisoning* has also been underestimated in the past and based on recent recorded cases it is calculated to be in the region of 1 mg F/kg body weight. This is less conservative than the estimate made by Duxbury et al.[19] in their review on fluoride toxicity.

The exact mechanism by which fluoride produces its toxic effect is still not known. In cases of minor acute poisoning, symptoms are salivation, nausea, vomiting and diarrhoea. These usually occur within an hour of ingestion. Consequently, if overdosage occurs as a result of topical fluoride application these symptoms may not be manifest until the patient has left the surgery. In cases of fatal poisoning, death occurs within 24 hours as a result of respiratory or cardiac failure.

Table 7.4 Toxicity of fluoride preparations (calculated for a 5-year-old child weighing 20 kg).

Fluoride agent	*Toxic doses of fluoride agents* — *Acute fluoride poisoning*	*Lethal*
APF solution or gel (1·23% F)	1·7 ml (1/3 tsp)	24 ml (1/4 cup)
Stannous fluoride solution (8·0% SnF_2)	1 ml (1/5 tsp)	14 ml (3 tsp)
Sodium fluoride varnish (2·26% F)	0·9 ml (1/5 tsp)	13 ml (2½ tsp)
Rinse (0·2% NaF)	22 ml (1/5 cup)	317 ml (3 cups)
Rinse (0·05% NaF)	88 ml (4/5 cup)	1268 ml (12½ cups)
Rinse concentrate (2·0% NaF)	2·2 ml (1/2 tsp)	32 ml (1/3 cup)
Tablets	20 tablets	286 tablets

1 cup = 100 ml, 1 teaspoon (tsp) = 5 ml.

Listed in *Table* 7.4 are some of the fluoride agents in use, the amount required to produce early toxic effects (1 mg/kg) and the acute lethal dose (14·28 mg/kg)—all in relation to the average 5-year-old child weighing about 20 kg (44 lb). It is apparent that as far as APF solutions and gels are concerned, as little as a third of a teaspoonful can produce toxic effects, while a quarter of a paper cupful can be lethal. Stannous fluoride solutions are used in higher concentration so that as little as a fifth of a teaspoonful can produce vomiting. On the other hand, it would take 20 × 1 mg F tablets to make a child vomit and 286 to kill.

If only a small quantity of fluoride is swallowed (below 5 mg F/kg body weight) the antidote is a large volume of milk. However, if quantities greater than 5 mg F/kg body weight have been ingested or if there is any doubt about the exact quantity consumed than it is advisable to refer the child to hospital where gastric lavage will probably be carried out. As fluoride is rapidly absorbed, speed is of the utmost importance.

7.10. SUMMARY

a. It is possible to reduce the susceptibility of teeth to caries progression by fluoride supplements.

b. Dental practitioners must be aware of the fluoride levels of local water supplies since no fluoride tablets or drops should be prescribed when the water contains more than 0·7 parts/10^6 F.

c. When fluoride tablets or drops are prescribed for the pre-school child, instructions should be given to limit the quantity of fluoridated toothpaste used to the size of a small pea, twice a day.

d. Frequent exposure of enamel to fluoride is necessary for the maximum caries-reducing effect.

e. The regular use of agents containing low concentrations of fluoride is more effective and safer than the irregular use of agents containing high concentrations of fluoride.

f. The caries-reducing effect of topical fluorides is greater in newly erupted teeth than in more mature teeth. Nevertheless, caries-prone adults do benefit from such treatment.

g. The choice of fluoride preparations ultimately depends on the age, cooperation and needs of the individual patient.

h. The use of fluorides in dental practice should always be combined with dietary advice and oral hygiene instruction.

REFERENCES

1. McKay F. S. (1916) An investigation into mottled teeth (1). *Dent. Cosmos* **58,** 477–484.
2. Churchill H. V. (1931) The occurrence of fluorides in some waters of the United States. *J. Ind. Eng. Chem.* **23,** 996–998.
3. Ainsworth N. J. (1933) Mottled teeth. *Br. Dent. J.* **60,** 233–250.
4. Dean H. T., Arnold F. A. and Evolve E. (1942) Domestic water and dental caries V, additional studies of the relation of fluoride domestic waters to dental caries experience in 4,425 white children aged 12–14 years, of 13 cities in 4 States. *Public Health Rep.* **65,** 1403–1408.
5. Murray J. J. and Rugg-Gunn A. (1982) *Fluorides in Caries Prevention.* Bristol, Wright.

6. Nikiforuk G. (1985) *Understanding Dental Caries, Vol. 1.* Basel, S. Karger, Chapter 4.
7. Isaac S., Brudevold F., Smith F. A. et al. (1958) The relation of fluoride in the drinking water to the distribution of fluoride in enamel. *J. Dent. Res.* **37,** 318–325.
8. Silverstone L. M., Johnson N. W., Hardie J. M. et al. (1984) *Dental Caries Aetiology, Pathology and Prevention.* London, Macmillan, Chapter 10.
9. Joyston-Bechal S. (1984) Fluoride supplementation in practice. *Dent. Update* **11,** 145–152.
10. Dowell T. B. and Joyston-Bechal S. (1981) Fluoride supplements—age related dosages. *Br. Dent. J.* **150,** 273–275.
11. Ekstrand J., Koch G., Lingfren L. E. et al. (1981) Pharmacokinetics of fluoride gels in children and adults. *Caries Res.* **15,** 213–220.
12. Speirs R. L. (1983) The value of prenatally administered fluoride. *Dent. Update* **10,** 43–51
13. Fejerskov O., Thylstrup A. and Larsen M. J. (1977) Clinical and structural features and possible pathogenic mechanisms of dental fluorosis. *Scand. J. Dent. Res.* **85,** 510–534.
14. Ekstrand J. (1977) Fluoride concentrations in saliva after single oral doses and their relation to plasma fluoride. *Scand. J. Dent. Res.* **85,** 16–17.
15. Ekstrand J. and Ehrnebo M. (1980) Absorbtion of fluoride from fluoride dentifrices. *Caries Res.* **14,** 96–102
16. Forest J. R. (1956) Caries experience and enamel defects in areas with different levels of fluoride in the drinking water. *Br. Dent. J.* **100,** 195–200
17. Small B. W. and Murray J. J. (1978) Enamel opacities; prevalence, classifications and aetiological considerations. *J. Dent.* **6,** 33–42.
18. Hodge H. C., Smith F. A. and Simmons J. H. (eds) (1965) *Fluorine Chemistry, Vol. 4.* London, Academic Press.
19. Duxbury A. J., Leach F. N. and Duxbury J. T. (1982) Acute fluoride toxicity. *Br. Dent. J.* **153,** 64–66.

CHAPTER 8

FISSURE SEALANTS

8.1. INTRODUCTION AND RATIONALE

Pits and fissures provide a sheltered environment in which dental plaque can develop. These areas are particularly susceptible to dental decay and are least benefitted by fluoride. Fissure sealants are materials designed to prevent pit and fissure caries. They are applied, mainly to the occlusal surfaces of the teeth, to obliterate the occlusal fissures, thus removing the sheltered environment in which caries may thrive.

8.2. HISTORICAL BACKGROUND

The problem of pit and fissure caries was recognized long ago. In the 1920s it was suggested that cavities should be prepared and filled with amalgam in all pits and fissures. This was called 'prophylactic odontotomy' and has been likened to justifying suicide with the argument that death comes to everyone sooner or later![1] However, this technique was a forerunner of today's sealant.

An alternative suggestion, also made in the 1920s, was that pits and fissures should be eradicated by widening them with small burs to produce rounded channels. However, although more conservative than prophylactic odontotomy, this interesting idea also involved the removal of healthy tooth structure. A number of workers tried to prevent the onset of decay by applying chemicals such as silver nitrate to the fissure system, trying to make the enamel more resistant to bacterial action. Attempts were also made to occlude the fissure system with black copper cement, but both this approach, and the use of silver nitrate were found to be ineffective in preventing caries.[2]

The advent of the fissure sealants as we know them today had to wait for the development of the acid-etch technique by Buonocore in 1955. This classic work described the application of phosphoric acid to enamel, to etch the tissue, creating porosities within it. When acrylic resin was then applied, the resin flowed into the holes in the enamel, thus bonding the material to the tooth. Subsequently a superior resin system was developed by Bowen at the National Bureau of Standards in America. Chemically, it is based on the product of bisphenol A and glycidyl methacrylate, commonly referred to as BIS-GMA or Bowen's resin. Most modern fissure sealants are based on Bowen's resin and are bonded to the enamel using the acid-etch technique.

8.3. THE ACID-ETCH TECHNIQUE

When 30–50 per cent phosphoric acid is applied for one minute to a clean enamel surface, two things happen. First of all, a small amount of enamel is dissolved (*Fig.* 8.1). About 8 μm of tissue is lost, which compares with 2–3 μm lost when teeth are polished with prophylactic paste (1 000 μm = 1 mm). In addition to this loss of tissue, porosities (about 50 μm deep) are produced in the enamel surface.

Three basic types of surface change have been described (*see Figs.* 8.2, 8.3 and 8.4). In the most common, type 1 etching pattern, prism core material is preferentially removed, leaving the prism peripheries relatively intact (*Fig.* 8.2). In the second, type 2 etching pattern, the reverse is observed. The peripheral regions of the prisms are removed preferentially, leaving prism cores relatively unaffected (*Fig.* 8.3). In the type 3 etching pattern, there is more haphazard effect not readily related to prism

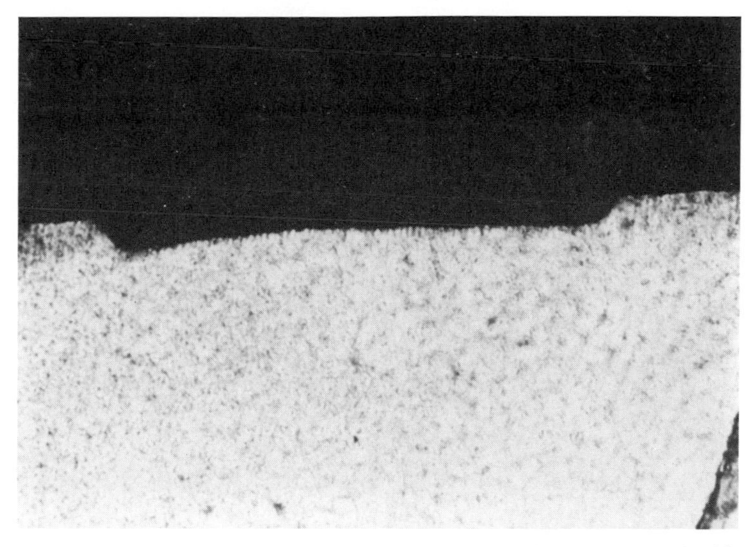

Fig. 8.1. A longitudinal ground section through an area of enamel exposed to 30 per cent phosphoric acid for 60 seconds. About 8 μm of enamel has been lost from the surface of the etched area. (Magnification × 500.)

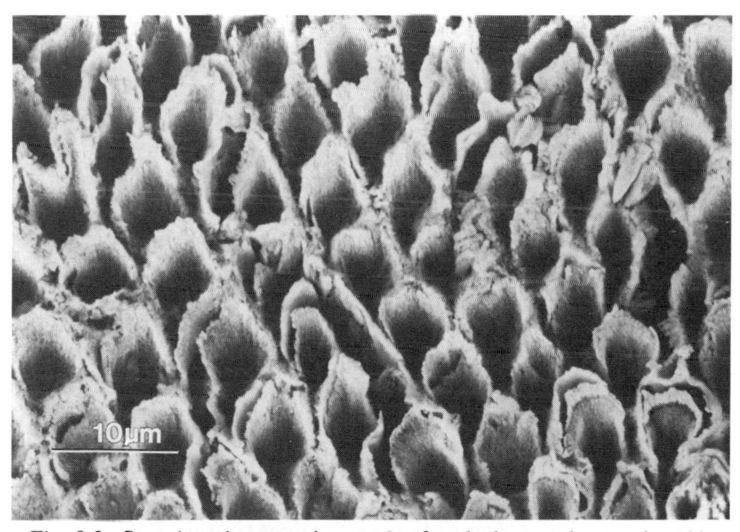

Fig. 8.2. Scanning electron micrograph of etched enamel, type 1 etching pattern. Prism core material is preferentially removed, leaving the prism periphery relatively intact (space bar = 10 μm). (By courtesy of Professor L. M. Silverstone.)

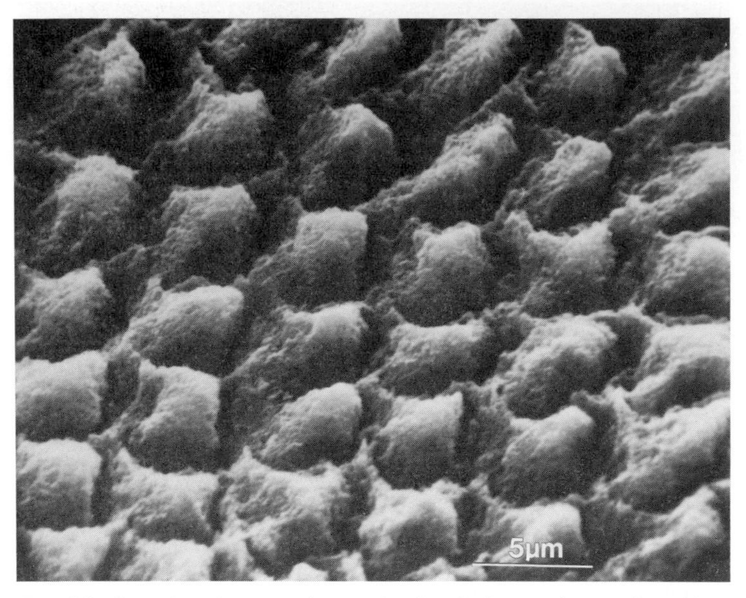

Fig. 8.3. Scanning electron micrograph of etched enamel, type 2 etching pattern. Peripheral regions of prisms removed preferentially, leaving prism cores relatively unaffected (space bar = 5 μm). (By courtesy of Professor L. M. Silverstone.)

morphology (*Fig.* 8.4). All three etching types can be found in a single sample of etched enamel.

The concentration of phosphoric acid has been chosen to be between 30 and 50 per cent to minimize loss of surface tissue but to produce porosities of maximum depth. Once the resin material is applied, it flows into the porosities where it polymerizes to form retentive tags (*Fig.* 8.5). This is the key to the success of acid-etch bonding since the tags mechanically attach the material to the enamel.

8.4. THE RESIN MATERIAL

The modern fissure sealant resins are based on Bowen's resin. Two types of resin material are available, those cured by exposure to light and those which set chemically.

Light-activated materials have the advantage that the operator has better control over the setting time but the disadvantage that extra expense is involved in purchasing and maintaining the light source. Polymerization of the early light-activated materials was initiated by ultraviolet light and one of the best known of these materials was called Nuvaseal (L. D. Caulk). In recent years visible light curing resin systems have become available. These

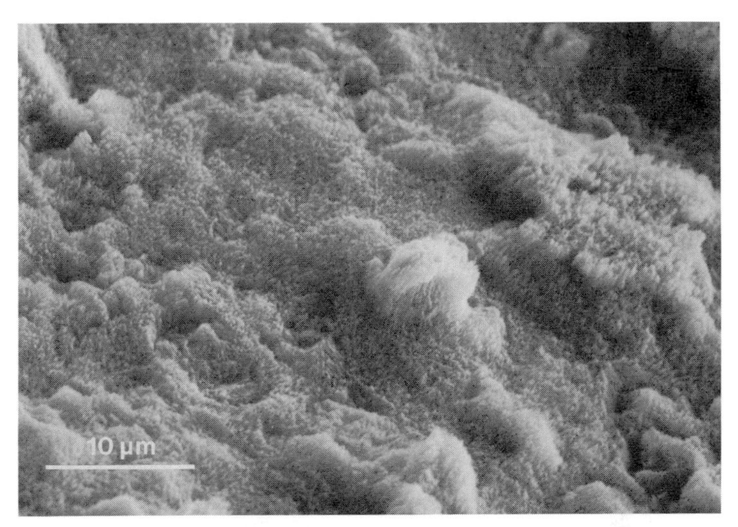

Fig. 8.4. Scanning electron micrograph of etched enamel, type 3 etching pattern showing a more haphazard effect not readily related to prism morphology (space bar = 10 μm). (By courtesy of Professor L. M. Silverstone.)

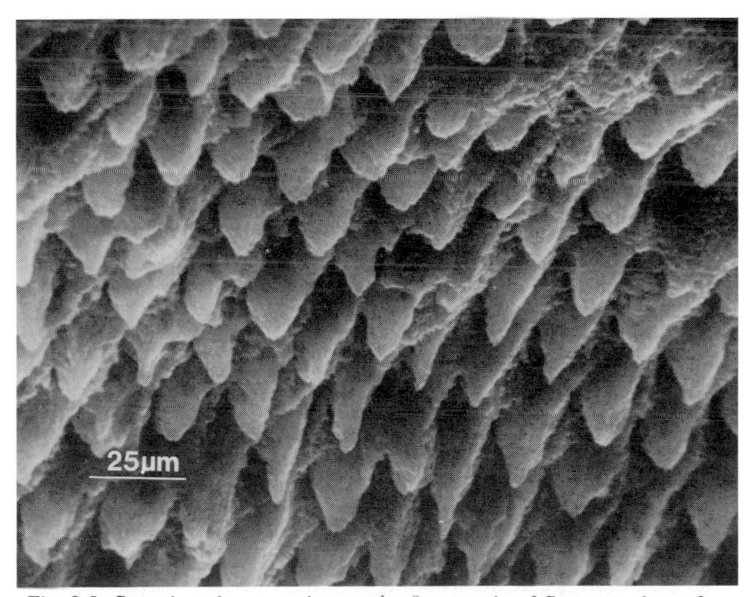

Fig. 8.5. Scanning electron micrograph of a sample of fissure sealant after demineralization of the adjacent enamel. The inner fitting surface of the resin shows tags approximately 30 μm long. (By courtesy of Professor L. M. Silverstone.)

visible light sources are able to penetrate greater depths of resin and may be safer as far as the operator is concerned. In the long term, exposure of the dentist's eyes to ultraviolet and possibly visible light may be damaging; thus it would seem prudent to wear eye protective dark glasses or to avoid staring directly at the light source when such glasses are not in use.

Chemical materials are naturally favoured by practitioners who wish to avoid the extra expense of buying the light source. Two particularly popular materials have been Delton (Johnson & Johnson Ltd) and Concise White Sealant System (3M Co.). The latter is of special interest because of its colour. Most sealants are difficult to detect clinically because the resin is translucent and takes up the colour of the underlying tooth. However, the Concise White Sealant System is coloured brilliant white, as its name suggests, which helps the dentist check its retention at recall appointments.

The early resins were all unfilled materials but in later years manufacturers started to incorporate fine glass filler particles in the material. They were thus very similar to composite resins which are also based on Bowen's resin but are heavily filled. The modern filled fissure sealant resins contain approximately 50 per cent of filler particles. These materials are less susceptible to abrasion than their unfilled counterparts and since wear of a fissure sealant will eventually lead to loss of the material, the new filled resins are to be preferred. Examples of modern filled fissure sealants cured by visible light are Nuva-cote and Prismashield (Caulk Co.). Estiseal (Kulzer GmbH) is a material produced in both a self-curing and visible light curing form.

8.5. CLINICAL TRIALS

Any new technique must always be carefully investigated in clinical trials, and an enormous number of these have now been undertaken demonstrating the efficacy of fissure sealants.[2, 3] The materials are usually tested in the first permanent molars where they are applied shortly after eruption of the teeth.

Trials have been designed to compare fissure sealing of one molar to no treatment of the contralateral molar in the same mouth. In addition, many trials have been designed to compare different sealant materials, again in the same mouth. In all these trials retention of the sealant has been a parameter that has been carefully measured since, to be effective, the sealant must be retained on the tooth. In addition, caries status has also been recorded.

Many of these trials have demonstrated excellent retention of the materials although the resin wears and is thus progressively lost from the tooth surface as time goes by. The loss of resin is most marked during the first 6 months but there is a further progressive loss. However, the lightly filled resins appear more abrasion resistant than their unfilled counterparts.

Retention for 10 years has been recorded, a figure that compares very favourably with the life of an amalgam restoration.

An interesting point to emerge from all the clinical trials is that there was considerable variation in the results obtained both with different materials and with different operators using the same material. This has important implications. First of all, some of the early materials were not particularly satisfactory. An example of this was a light-cured material which was subsequently marketed as Alphaseal (Amalgamated Dental Ltd). When the experimental version of this material was tested clinically, there was only 2·3 per cent retention of the sealant at 1 year. Subsequently, laboratory studies demonstrated that the material did not set at depth. This emphasizes the importance of clinical trials as well as laboratory studies and the need for dentists to keep abreast of the literature so that patients may benefit as more is learnt about materials and techniques.

Another interesting and important observation was that different operators obtained different results with the same materials. This must mean that the manner in which a material is handled is critical to its subsequent clinical performance. Laboratory research has done much to establish the aspects of clinical technique that are critical and these will be discussed fully in section 8.7.

8.6. CLINICAL INDICATIONS

8.6.1. Permanent Teeth

Since caries in pits and fissures is difficult to diagnose in its early stage, the dentist may decide to fissure seal susceptible teeth as soon after eruption as possible. First and second permanent molars are obvious candidates, but while some dentists may decide to seal the fissures of all newly erupted teeth as a routine, many others will use some of the following criteria when deciding whether or not to fissure seal.

a. Is the tooth newly erupted? A tooth which has been in the mouth for many years without becoming carious is unlikely to need a fissure sealant.

b. Can the tooth be isolated from salivary contamination? Salivary contamination during fissure sealant placement is the most common cause of failure of a sealant. If this occurs and the patient is lucky, the sealant will fall off and there will be no permanent harm. However, if the sealant is partly retained but leaking, caries can progress beneath it, safe from salivary protection, fluoride ions and detection by the dentist (*see* section 8.8). Thus good isolation from saliva is an essential part of the clinical technique. The only reliable method of isolation is the use of a rubber dam.

c. Does the child show some evidence of caries in other teeth? Signs of caries or extractions elsewhere in the mouth indicate caries risk and will favour the use of sealants.

d. Does the tooth have a deep fissure pattern that will be difficult to keep clean or a coalesced fissure pattern of shallow rounded grooves unlikely to decay?

e. Is the patient's oral hygiene poor? Although oral hygiene and caries status are not well correlated in clinical trials, poor oral hygiene may indicate a lack of dental awareness and cooperation.

f. Has the dentist reason to believe the patient's diet contains much sugar? Dietary analysis is important in assessing caries risk.

g. If facilities are available for microbiological tests, *Streptococcus mutans* and lactobacillus counts may assist in predicting caries risk.

h. Does the dentist anticipate that the patient might be difficult to manage when carrying out restorative dentistry? A non-operative procedure, like fissure sealing, may demand a little less patient cooperation.

i. Does the patient belong to a group in which it is of particular importance to prevent dental caries, e.g. patients with cleft palates or bleeding diatheses such as haemophilia?

The problems of diagnosing occlusal caries were discussed in Chapter 4. Sharp eyes, dry clean teeth and good bitewing radiographs are essential. The early occlusal lesion is not readily seen but progression may be rapid, cavitation occurring in less than 1 year. The lesion results in gross undermining of enamel. For all these reasons a 'wait and watch' approach is not advocated with fissure caries. If the caries risk is assessed as high, a fissure sealant is indicated as part of a total preventive programme.

8.6.2. Deciduous Teeth

Deciduous molar teeth are not fissure sealed as often as permanent molar teeth. The main indication for fissure sealing is finding caries elsewhere in the dentition, i.e. caries risk is high.

8.7. CLINICAL TECHNIQUE

8.7.1. Isolation

Isolation is probably the most critical step with regard to the success or failure of the sealant. If saliva blocks the pores created by etching the bond will be weakened. A rubber dam is the most predictable method of isolation and is preferred to the use of cotton wool rolls and a saliva ejector. The latter are difficult to use effectively because after etching the teeth must be thoroughly washed. This inevitably soaks the cotton wool rolls which must then be changed. While this is being done, it is all too easy to drop saliva over the etched tooth surface and this contamination will ruin the bond of the sealant to the enamel.

When a rubber dam is applied for fissure sealing only the tooth to be treated need be isolated.[4] Since a rubber dam clamp will be required, and clamps can be uncomfortable, a small amount of local anaesthetic may be

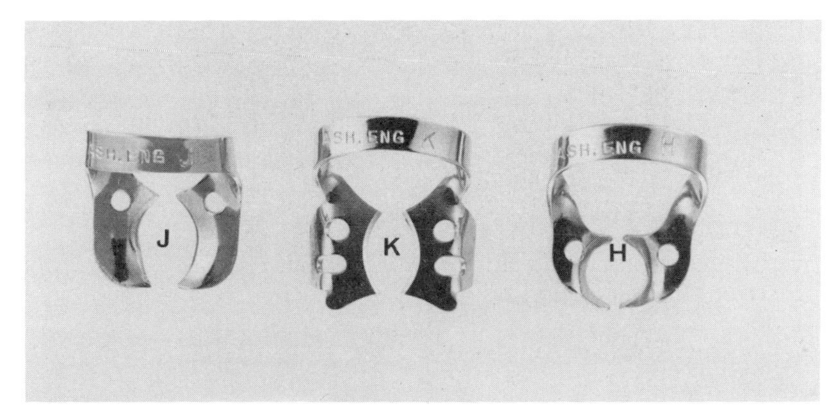

Fig. 8.6. A selection of rubber dam clamps. Clamps J and K are bland; H is retentive; J and H are wingless; K is winged.

infiltrated buccally and lingually to the tooth to be treated. Alternatively topical anaesthetic may be liberally applied to the gingival margin. A clamp of suitable size is selected and tried on the tooth, placing it just coronal to the gingival margin. Where the maximum convexity of the tooth is subgingival, a retentive rubber dam clamp is required, but where the tooth is fully erupted, a bland clamp should be chosen (*see Fig.* 8.6). Floss should be attached to the holes of the clamp so that the dentist can retrieve it should the clamp fracture across the bow (*Fig.* 8.7*a*).

If the clamp is postioned before applying the rubber, it is convenient to select a wingless clamp for molar teeth (*Fig.* 8.7*a*). Having placed the clamp on the tooth, the floss is threaded through the punched and lubricated hole in the rubber dam (*Fig.* 8.7*b*). The dental surgery assistant then gently pulls on the floss as the dentist slides the rubber over the bow of the clamp, one side (*Fig.* 8.7*c*) and then the other side. Should the clamp fracture across the bow, the dental surgery assistant would be able to retrieve the pieces by pulling on the floss.

An alternative technique is to apply clamp and rubber simultaneously. In this case a winged clamp must be chosen (*see Fig.* 8.6.) and the wings engaged in the lubricated hole (*Fig.* 8.8*a*). Clamp and rubber are then applied simultaneously. The dental surgery assistant should gently retract the rubber so that the dentist can see the tooth clearly (*Fig.* 8.8*b*). A disadvantage of this method is that the dentist cannot see the gingival margin when placing the clamp. Once the clamp is in position a flat plastic instrument is used to disengage the rubber from the wings of the clamp (*Fig.* 8.8*c*). If this step is omitted, saliva will leak around the tooth.

A piece of soft material, such as paper towelling, in which a mouth hole has been cut, is now placed between the rubber and the patient's face to

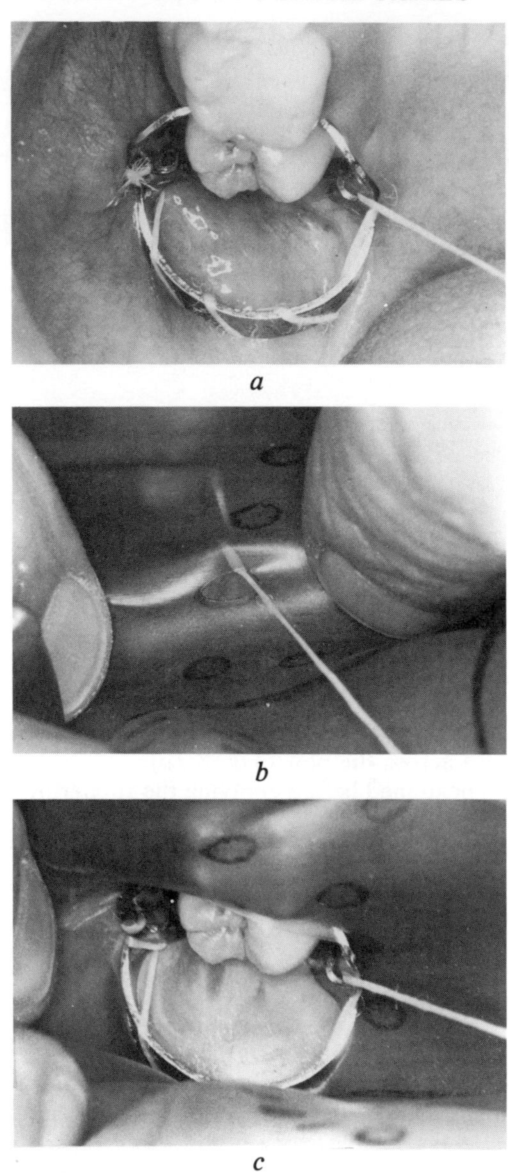

Fig. 8.7. *a.* A wingless clamp in position on 7 . Floss has been attached to the holes of the clamp so that the dentist can retrieve it should the clamp fracture across the bow. *b.* The floss is now threaded through the punched and lubricated hole in the rubber dam. *c.* The dentist now slides the rubber over the bow of the clamp, one side and then the other side. The dental surgery assistant gently pulls on the floss as the rubber is placed.

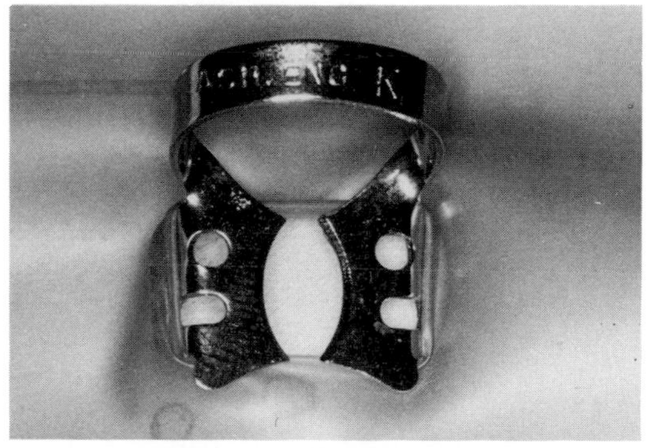

a

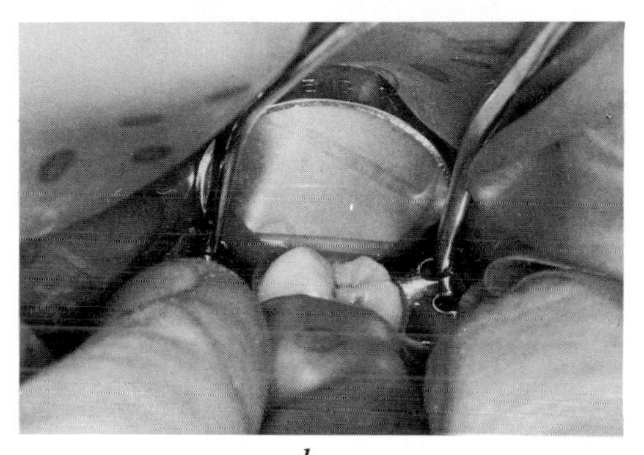

b

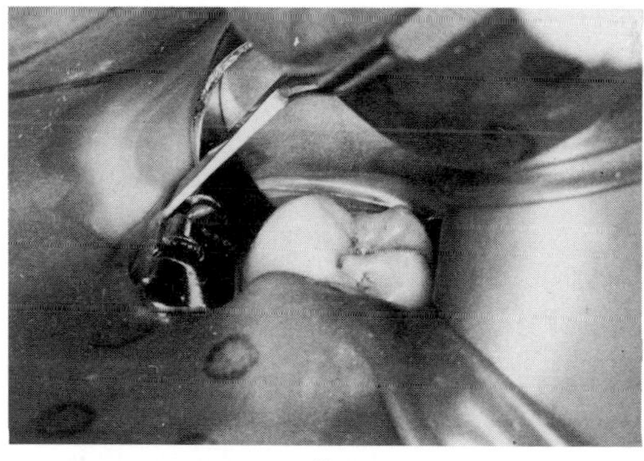

c

Fig. 8.8. *a.* A winged rubber dam clamp engaged in the lubricated hole in the rubber. *b.* Clamp and rubber are being placed on the tooth simultaneously. The dental surgery assistant should gently retract the rubber so that the dentist can see the tooth clearly. *c.* A flat plastic instrument is used to disengage the rubber from the wings of the clamp.

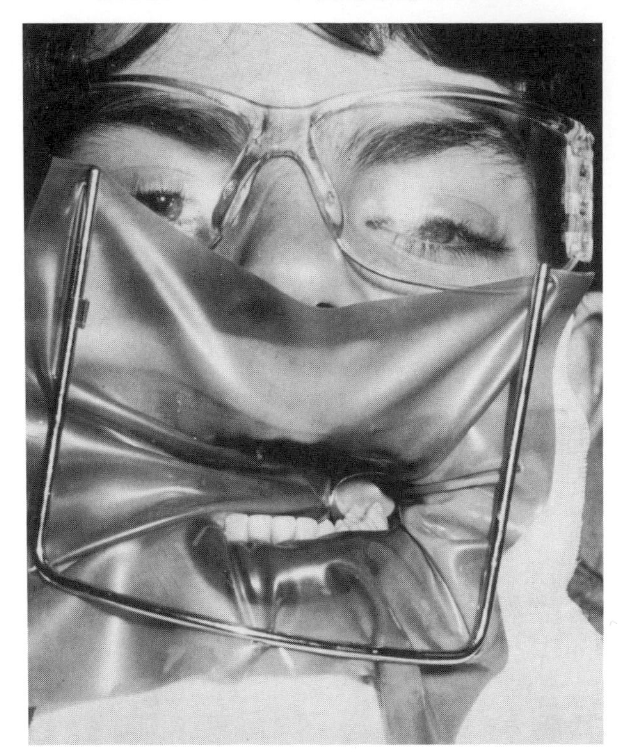

Fig. 8.9. A rubber dam in position. Note a soft towel separates the rubber from the face. The rubber may be trimmed to avoid contact with the nose, although this was not done in this case because the patient was comfortable.

prevent the uncomfortable feeling of rubber against the face. Finally the frame is positioned (*Fig.* 8.9).

8.7.2. Cleaning the Teeth

The tooth surface to be etched and sealed must be thoroughly cleaned with a rotating brush and a pumice and water slurry. Oil-based mixtures of pumice should not be used as these may interfere with etching. The pumice is washed away with a blast of water and air from the 3 in 1 syringe, then a sharp probe is dragged through the fissure system. This will remove some of the deeper plaque the brush cannot reach. The tooth is then washed again and thoroughly dried.

8.7.3. Etching

The phosphoric acid etchant is supplied by the manufacturer in the form of either a colourless liquid or a coloured gel. The gel is preferred as it is much easier to control. The etchant is applied over the whole occlusal surface and any lingual or buccal surface where grooves require sealing (*Fig.* 8.10*a*). Etching the entire occlusal surface avoids the danger of covering an unetched surface with sealant and thus inviting leakage. The acid can be applied with either a tiny pledget of cotton wool, a tiny gauze sponge or a small brush. Alternatively a fine syringe may be used to apply the gel etchant. As soon as the complete area to be etched is covered with acid, the time is noted, and the tooth enamel is etched for 60 seconds. When acid is used in the liquid form, fresh solution can be dabbed on the surfaces during etching but care should be taken to treat the enamel surface very carefully. Rubbing the cotton wool pledget or sponge on the surface during acid application may damage the fragile enamel latticework being formed.

8.7.4. Washing

After 60 seconds the acid is washed away. Initially a water spray is used from the 3 in 1 syringe to remove most of the acid. After approximately 5 seconds of spraying water, the air button is also pressed, forming a strong water-air spray which should be played over the etched surface for at least 15–20 seconds. If gels are used, the wash time should be doubled to at least 30 seconds to ensure removal of the gel and reaction products. During the washing phase all excess water is removed with the aspirator by the dental surgery assistant.

8.7.5. Drying the Etched Enamel

The tooth surface is now thoroughly dried with air from the 3 in 1 syringe. The drying phase is most important since any moisture on the etched surface will hinder penetration of the resin into the enamel. A minimum of 15 seconds drying is recommended. At this stage the etched area should appear matt and white (*Fig.* 8.10*b*). It is good practice to check that the airline is not contaminated by water or oil by blowing it at a clean glass surface. Any moisture or oil coming from the airline will cause the technique to fail.

With a rubber dam in position, there should be no danger of salivary contamination of the etched surface. If this does occur, however, it is essential to re-etch the enamel because the saliva will block the pores which are essential for optimal bonding.

8.7.6. Mixing the Resin

A light-cured resin material does not require mixing. A chemically cured resin (self-curing resin) has two components which are gently mixed together to avoid incorporating air bubbles.

8.7.7. Sealant Application

A small disposable brush or applicator, supplied by the manufacturer, is used to apply the sealant to the pits and fissures and up the etched cuspal

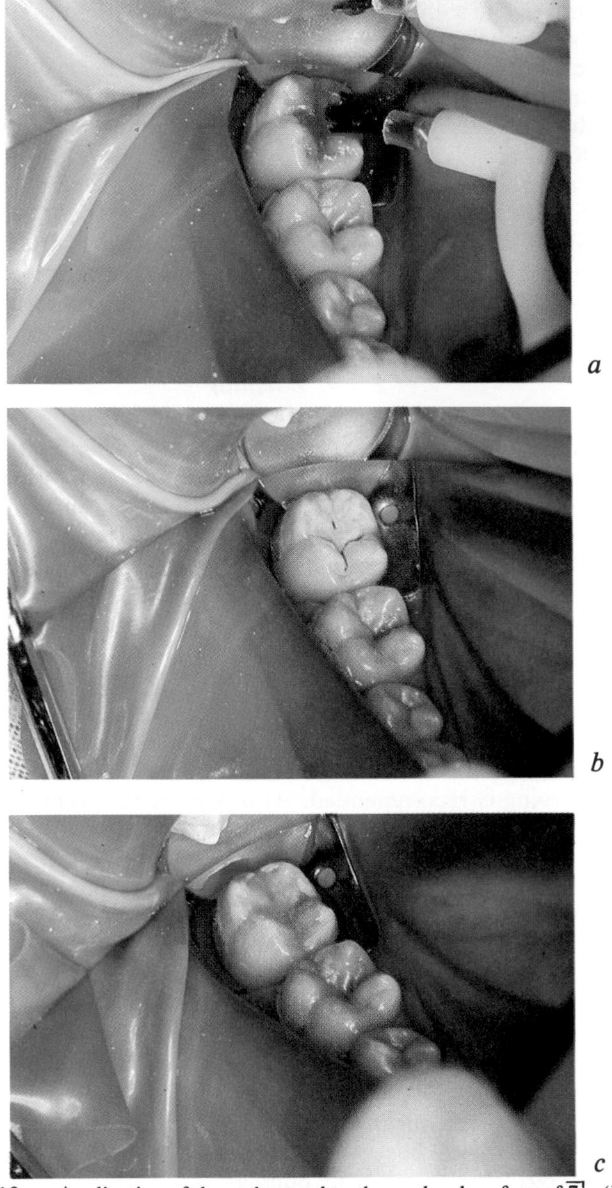

Fig. 8.10. *a.* Application of the etchant gel to the occlusal surface of $\overline{7|}$. (By courtesy of Dr G. Roberts.) *b.* The dried etched area on $\overline{7|}$ appears matt and white. (By courtesy of Dr G. Roberts.) *c.* The completed fissure sealant. Note it has been applied within the etched area to ensure marginal seal. (By courtesy of Dr G. Roberts.)

slopes. If a light-cured material has been chosen, the light should be placed directly over the sealant, but should not touch it. The sealant is exposed to the light for a full 60 seconds to cure it. It is essential to time this carefully as an incompletely cured material is doomed to failure. In addition, with a molar tooth, the light source should be directed at the distal part of the occlusal surface for 60 seconds and then moved to the mesial aspect for a further 60 seconds. Any buccal or palatal groove or pit should be similarly cured with the light source directly over it.

Most chemically cured sealants polymerize in one to three minutes and the manufacturer's instructions should be consulted to check the setting time of the particular material chosen. The outer surface layer of any sealant will not polymerize, due to the inhibiting effect of oxygen in the atmosphere. Thus the sealant will always appear to have a greasy film after polymerization (*Fig.* 8.10*c*).

8.7.8. Checking Occlusion

The rubber dam is now removed and occlusion checked with articulating paper. While it was considered acceptable to allow any high spots to be abraded away when unfilled fissure sealants were used, with the new filled materials it is wiser to reduce high spots by grinding with a small round diamond stone in a conventional handpiece.

8.8. RECALL AND REASSESSMENT

It cannot be stressed too strongly that a fissure sealed tooth is not immune from caries. A well bonded sealant will prevent decay but a leaking sealant is a recipe for disaster. For this reason, fissure sealed teeth must be reviewed with the same care as unfilled or restored surfaces. This means that every 6 months the teeth must be isolated with cotton wool rolls and dried. The sealant should then be checked visually. Any discoloration of the sealant, the margin of the sealant or the underlying enamel must be viewed with suspicion as this may indicate leakage. A careful check should be made for partial or complete loss of the material. Coloured and filled resins are easier to see than the colourless and unfilled materials. However, the latter have the advantage that caries beneath them can be detected as a brown discoloration. In addition to a visual check, some operators advocate the use of a Briault probe to check that the sealant is firmly attached to the tooth and cannot be lifted off.

Finally, bitewing radiographs of sealed teeth must be carefully checked for signs of caries. Operative intervention is called for if caries is seen.

A sealant which is partly lost or one where a margin is discoloured can be repaired by removing as much of the old sealant as possible, re-etching and applying fresh sealant. Provided a clean surface is produced, new sealant will bond to the old material although this bond is not as strong as the original intact material.

8.9. ASSESSMENT OF RISKS ASSOCIATED WITH SEALANTS

Two questions are frequently raised concerning sealants and the acid-etch technique.

8.9.1. What Happens to Etched Areas that are Not Covered by Sealant?

These areas remineralize from the saliva and there is no evidence that they are subsequently more prone to caries. Some operators cover the sealant/etched enamel junction with fluoride varnish.

8.9.2. What Happens if a Carious Lesion is Inadvertently Sealed Over?

This is a very important question because fissure caries is notoriously difficult to diagnose and fissure sealants are probably frequently placed on fissures which would show early lesions if they were examined histologically. Fortunately, clinical research suggests that if a tooth with early occlusal caries is treated with a fissure sealant, there is reasonable hope of a favourable outcome.[5] Where the sealant has remained intact, it has been shown that caries has not progressed. There is a decrease in the number of viable organisms and the metabolic activity of the remaining bacteria is reduced. This seems logical, since the bacteria are now cut off from their source of nutriment.

Thus the conscientious practitioner may be encouraged to adopt the maxim 'when in doubt, seal' rather than the alternative, 'when in doubt, cut'. Another approach is to enter such doubtful areas operatively with small burs, remove caries and use posterior composite resins to restore the defect and to seal the remaining fissure system. This is called a 'preventive resin restoration' and is discussed again in Chapter 10.

It is interesting to speculate that the time may come when it is acceptable to fissure seal relatively large lesions, cutting them off from the oral environment and thus arresting the disease. The authors would not currently advocate this approach, preferring to restore such teeth conventionally rather than risk a leaking sealant which could result in rapid pulp exposure.

8.10. THE COST-EFFECTIVENESS OF SEALANTS

Some attempts have been made to assess the cost-effectiveness of sealants. If every tooth with an occlusal surface were to be fissure sealed, fissure sealing would become more expensive than the alternative approach which is the restoration of carious teeth. However, this 'blunderbuss' approach would not be a correct use for sealants because not all teeth are going to decay. Thus prescription of sealants must be based on an assessment of caries risk.

If fissure sealants were only to be used on first permanent molars, soon after eruption of these teeth, the procedure would probably be 'cost-effective'. However, if caries risk is correctly assessed, not all these teeth will need to be fissure sealed. In a population with a falling caries rate preventive efforts must be targeted at those most in need.

In addition, the value of a successful sealant must not be costed in terms of clinical time and materials alone. The technique is atraumatic in contrast to operative dentistry. Unfortunately, research has shown that placing a restoration in a tooth can start a restorative cycle where restorations tend to be removed and replaced every 5–10 years with a consequent increase in size of the cavity. Eventually the tooth structure is so weakened that a crown is required and a failed crown may lead to extraction.

8.11. GLASS-IONOMER CEMENTS

In recent years the use of a glass-ionomer cement as a fissure sealant has been tried. This material contains aluminosilicate glass and polyacrylic acid and was the first permanent restorative material to be chemically adhesive to enamel and dentine. Etching of enamel is not required, but organic debris is removed using a special conditioner (polyacrylic acid) supplied with the material. This conditioning ensures a clean surface to receive the bond. An interesting feature of glass-ionomer cement is that it contains available fluoride, which may exert a cariostatic effect. To date there have been insufficient clinical trials on this technique to recommend its use with certainty. However, it will be interesting to follow the development of this group of materials.

REFERENCES

1. Simonsen R. J. (1978) *Clinical Applications of the Acid Etch Technique.* Chicago, Quintessence, Chapter 2.
2. Murray J. J. (1983) *The Prevention of Dental Disease.* Oxford, Oxford University Press, Chapter 5.
3. Stephen K. W. (1984) Fissure sealants—then, now and the future. In: *Cariology Today. Int. Congr. Zurich.* Basel, S. Karger, pp. 301–307.
4. Kidd E. A. M. (1983) Rubber dam—a reappraisal. *Dent. Update* **10,** 233–245.
5. Elderton R. J. (1985) Management of early dental caries in fissures with fissure sealant. *Br. Dent. J.* **158,** 254–258.

CHAPTER 9

PREVENTION OF CARIES BY PLAQUE CONTROL

9.1. INTRODUCTION[1]

Caries is a disease in which bacterial plaque interacts with the diet and the resistance of the host. There is no doubt that without plaque no caries would be initiated. Consequently one method of preventing caries is to try to control the deposition of plaque on the tooth surface, either by preventing its formation or by removing it at regular intervals.

There are two different approaches in the control of plaque for the prevention of caries.

9.1.1. Treatment Based on the 'Non-specific Plaque Hypothesis'

According to this hypothesis all plaque is potentially cariogenic, i.e. caries is the result of a non-specific infection. If this is true it follows that the main difference, as far as plaque is concerned, between a caries-inactive individual and an individual with rampant caries must lie only in the quantity present. Consequently, there would be no need to identify individuals at risk by using any bacteriological tests. It also follows that since everyone forms plaque daily, the whole population should be motivated to perform meticulous daily oral hygiene. Together with dietary advice and the use of fluorides this approach has been used in the last three decades with partial success.

9.1.2. Treatment Based on the 'Specific Plaque Hypothesis'

The advocates of this treatment philosophy suggest that plaque is not always cariogenic and that only certain plaques colonized by specific microorganisms are responsible for dental decay. Indeed, there is evidence that the bacterial composition of plaque varies from site to site within the same mouth as well as from individual to individual. It has been proposed by Loesche[1] in 1982 that, bacteriologically, at least three broad categories of plaque can be recognized: non-disease associated plaque, caries associated plaque and periodontal disease associated plaque. A summary of these types of plaque and their effects on the oral cavity, as suggested by Loesche, is shown in *Fig.* 9.1.

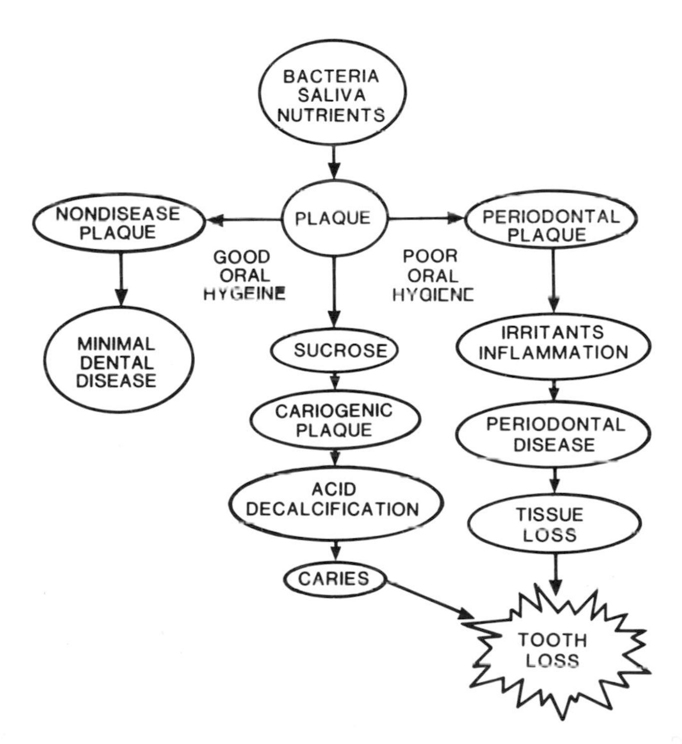

Fig. 9.1. A summary of the types of plaque and their effects on the oral cavity from Loesche (1982).[1]

The classic studies by Keyes (1960) and Fitzgerald and Keyes (1960) on germ-free animals showed that plaque dominated by *Streptococcus mutans* and lactobaccilli is responsible for dental caries. On the other hand, plaque which is not dominated by these microorganisms may be associated with a low caries prevalence.

Treatment based on the Specific Plaque Hypothesis begins by identifying individuals at risk with the aid of bacteriological tests. This is followed by a combination of dietary control (*see* Chapter 6), mechanical plaque control and the possible use of antimicrobial agents to suppress *S. mutans* in particular. Such treatment should, theoretically, result in the development of plaque which is largely composed of non-cariogenic organisms such as *S. sanguis* and *S. mitis* and only a low proportion of *S. mutans*.

Although there is no doubt that *S. mutans* is the most important microorganism implicated in caries, the microbial ecology of the mouth is highly complex. It is possible that strains of *S. mutans* may vary in their virulence and that other oral bacteria which are capable of producing acids from the fermentation of dietary carbohydrates may also be capable of initiating caries. Nevertheless, a microbiological examination in association with clinical criteria (*see* Chapter 4.4) may be a valuable tool in assessing the treatment needs of the patient.

Research efforts in plaque control have been generally directly along the following lines:

a. Mechanical removal of plaque.
b. Chemical methods to inhibit plaque formation or to eliminate specific bacteria and their products within plaque.
c. Immunological methods.

These three methods of controlling plaque in the prevention of caries will be discussed, wherever possible, in relation to the two treatment philosophies outlined.

9.2. MECHANICAL REMOVAL OF PLAQUE

9.2.1. Seeing Plaque: Disclosing Agents and Mirrors

In order to learn how to remove plaque effectively it is helpful for the patient to see where it is present. Since plaque is translucent and has a colour similar to teeth, it must be stained in order to be seen clearly (*see Fig.* 1.5*a* and *b*). Liquids, tablets and capsules containing erythrosin or vegetable dyes are used to stain plaque and are called 'disclosing agents'. Once a patient has been taught to identify plaque, the disclosing agent should be applied after toothbrushing so that areas where oral hygiene is inadequate can be seen easily. However, this will only be possible if the bathroom mirror used at home by the patient is well illuminated and a mouth mirror is also used. An inexpensive magnifying shaving mirror together with a disposable mouth mirror (*Fig.* 9.2) are invaluable aids for

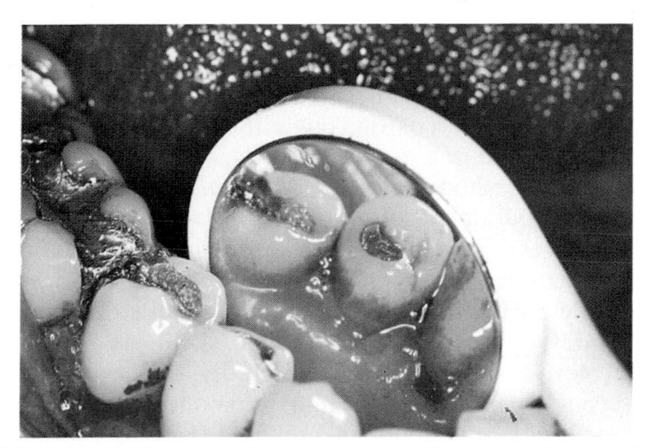

Fig. 9.2. A disposable mouth mirror allows the patient to see plaque on lingual and interproximal areas.

effective oral hygiene. When adequate lighting is a problem a mirror-light combination is a good solution.

9.2.2. Toothbrushes

Toothbrushes vary widely in shape and size of the head, the material, texture and arrangement of filaments as well as in the size and shape of the handles. However, at present nearly all toothbrushes available are multitufted with nylon filaments. Attempts have been made to establish the relative importance of the other variables in design but the results have been inconclusive. This is not surprising since the efficiency of a toothbrush in removing plaque is, for the most part, dependent on the care the subject exercises and to a very minor degree on the type of brush and method of brushing. Any toothbrush which allows a particular patient to reach all tooth surfaces easily and comfortably is acceptable although a medium brush with a small head is generally recommended. However, it is particularly important that brushes are replaced regularly, at least every 3 months or sooner if the filaments become permanently bent. A brush which shows such signs of wear cannot clean effectively. Although there is considerable variation in manual dexterity, most healthy individuals can be taught to clean their teeth effectively, provided they are sufficiently motivated. However, for the physically handicapped, where manual dexterity is limited, an electric toothbrush is very helpful.

9.2.3. Methods of Toothbrushing

Various methods of toothbrushing have been advocated and classified according to the type of motion performed by the brush:

a. The 'Scrub' method is performed by using a *horizontal* scrubbing motion and is usually recommended for children.

b. The 'Roll' or 'Rolling Stroke' method is carried out by pointing the filaments apically and then *rolling* or rotating them from the gingival margin to the occlusal or incisal edges of the teeth.

c. The 'Fones'' method is carried out with the teeth held in occlusion and the brush revolved in a *circular* motion.

d. The 'Leonard' method advocates a *vertical* stroke, brushing upper and lower teeth separately.

e. In the 'Charters'' and 'Bass' methods a *vibratory* motion is used.

Comparative studies of the effectiveness of these various methods of brushing provide conflicting and inconclusive results. This is because the subjects themselves contribute variables such as ability to follow instructions, motivation and manual dexterity that are hard to control. However, even when professional dental personnel were used in a study to compare three different methods of brushing (Charters', Scrub and Roll methods), the results were inconclusive. It would seem, therefore, that it does not matter which method is used as long as plaque is removed effectively without trauma to the gingival tissues. Ultimately the choice of method depends on the dexterity of the individual patient. Since the vibratory methods (Charters' and Bass) are the most commonly recommended they will be described in more detail.

The Charters' method (*see Fig.* 9.3)

The brush is held with the filaments *pointing towards the occlusal* plane and then applied to the teeth at an angle of 45° to this plane. The brush is pressed so that the filaments are flexed and the tips forced between the teeth. It is then vibrated by a rotary movement of the handle, keeping the

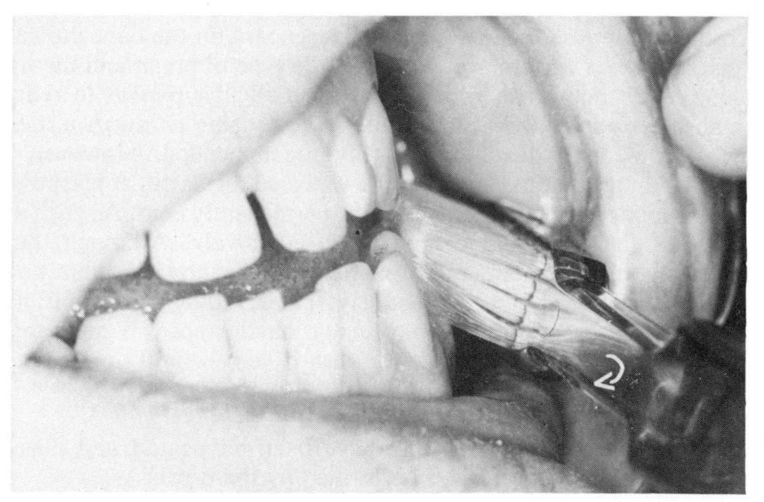

Fig. 9.3. The Charters' method of toothbrushing. Note the angulation of the bristles against the tooth surface.

tips of the bristles in position. This method of brushing is advocated in patients with open interdental spaces which facilitate the penetration of the brush filaments.

The Bass method (*see Fig.* 9.4)

The brush is held so that the filaments are directed *apically* and then placed against the gingival margin at an angle of 45° to the long axis of the tooth. The brush is then vibrated in an anterior–posterior direction. In order to clean the lingual surfaces of the upper and lower anterior teeth the brush has to be turned into a vertical position, using the bristles at the 'toe' of the brush to obtain proper access to the gingival area of the teeth.

The Bass method is effective in removing plaque adjacent to and directly below the gingival margin. Since the filaments of the brush are directed towards the gingival tissues and may be potentially damaging a hard brush must not be used with this method.

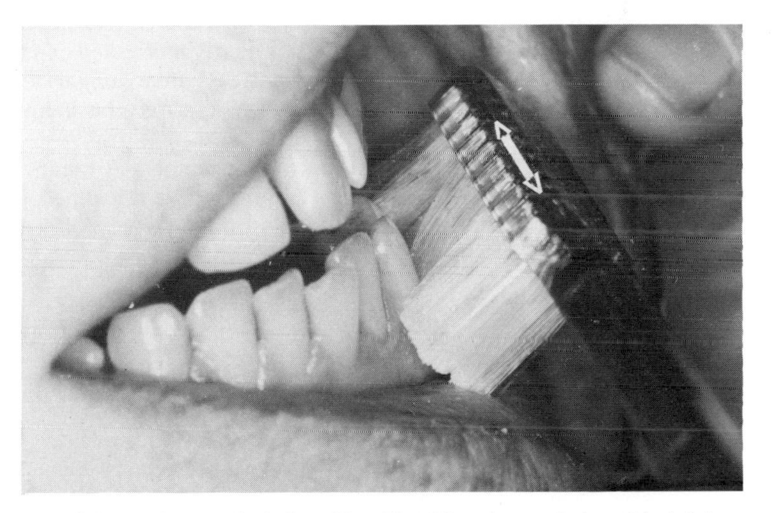

Fig. 9.4. The Bass method of toothbrushing. Note the angulation of the bristles against the tooth surface and the direction of the vibratory motion.

9.2.4. Interdental Cleaning

Approximal surfaces and areas where teeth are malaligned cannot be reached with an ordinary toothbrush. Consequently additional aids such as dental floss or tape, woodsticks, single-tufted brushes or interdental brushes may be required for these areas. Choice will depend on the shape of the interdental area and the dexterity of the individual.

Dental Floss or Tape

In a young and healthy mouth where the interdental papillae fill the interdental spaces, the use of dental floss or tape is the method of choice for interproximal cleaning. No differences have been found in cleansing potential between waxed and unwaxed floss although unwaxed floss tends to fray more readily.

It is necessary to teach the patient the correct technique for using floss, otherwise damage to the gingival tissues is likely. The technique is illustrated in *Figs.* 9.5 and 9.6. The fingers holding the floss should not be more than 15 mm apart. The floss should be guided slowly through the contact point and then wrapped around the interproximal surface of each tooth in turn. A sawing motion along the surface is then used to remove plaque. The index fingers of both hands are usually used to control the floss when the lower teeth are cleaned (*Fig.* 9.5). For the upper teeth it is recommended that the index finger of one hand and the thumb of the other hand are used (*Fig.* 9.6). A clean section of floss should be used for each interproximal space since it may be possible to transfer microorganisms from one site to another. Patients who are sufficiently motivated can usually learn to floss adequately although some patients take longer to grasp the technique. In such patients patent floss holders may be helpful (*see Fig.* 9.7).

'Super' floss (*see also Fig.* 9.7) is specially designed to clean under bridgework. A section of the floss, about 12 cm long, is thickened with a foamlike material and when threaded under a bridge is very effective in removing plaque (*Fig.* 9.8).

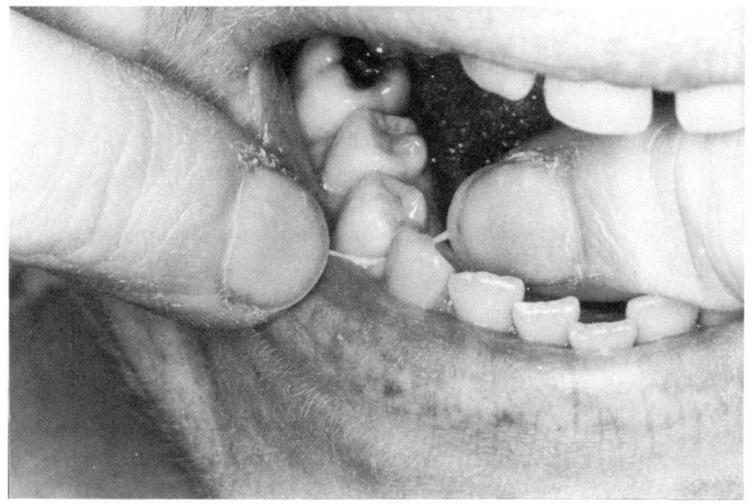

Fig. 9.5. The use of dental floss for interproximal cleaning of the lower teeth. Two index fingers are used to control the floss.

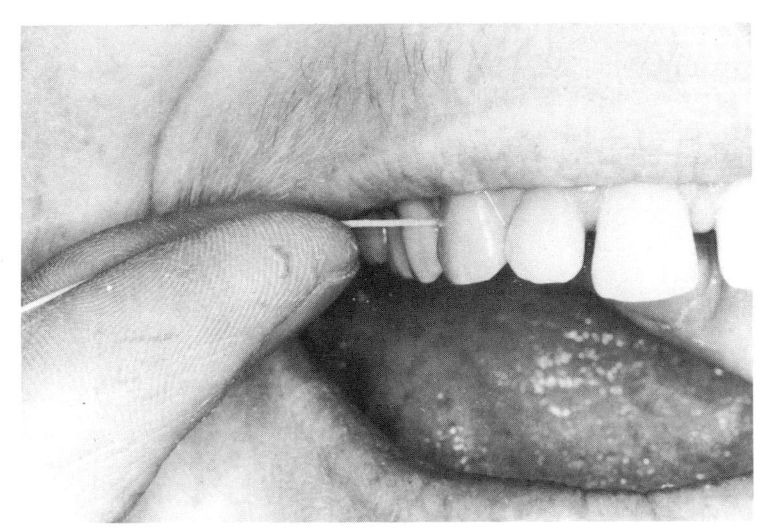

Fig. 9.6. The use of dental floss for interproximal cleaning of the upper teeth. The floss is controlled by the index finger of one hand and the thumb of the other.

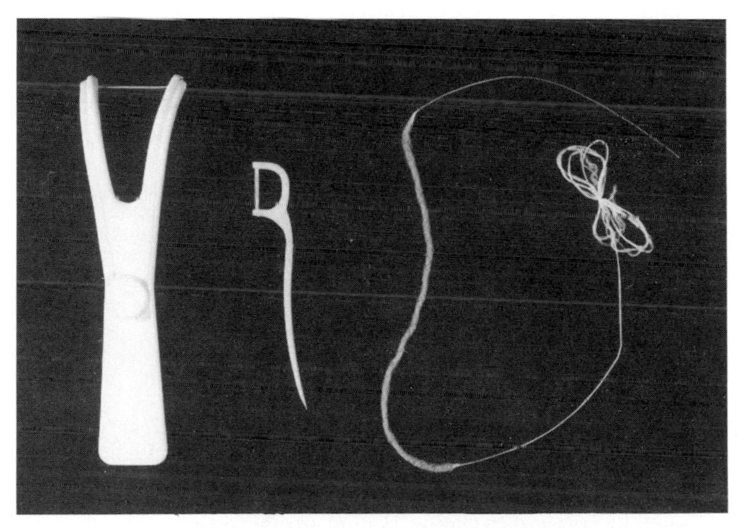

Fig. 9.7. Floss holders and 'Super' floss.

Woodsticks

When there is recession of the interdental papillae and consequently interdental spaces are present, woodsticks can be used for interproximal cleaning instead of dental floss.

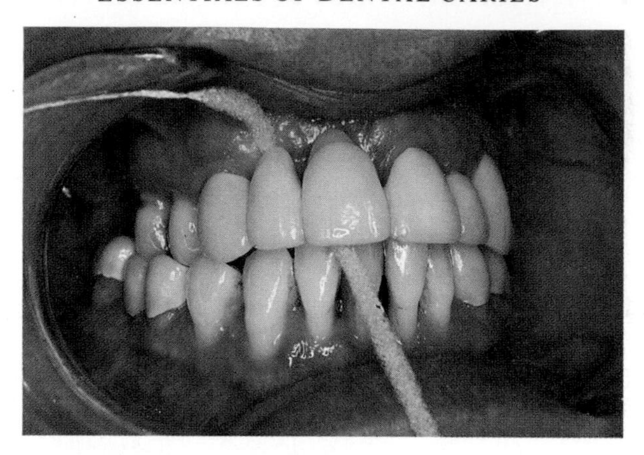

Fig. 9.8. The use of 'Super' floss to remove plaque under a bridge.

Woodsticks are made of soft wood and are triangular in cross-section so that they fit the interdental space. The base of the wedge is applied to the gingival border of the interdental area with the tip pointing towards the occlusal plane (*Fig.* 9.9). The interproximal surfaces are then cleaned by moving the woodstick in and out, applying pressure on each side of the embrasure in turn. In order to prevent the use of excessive force and to steady the fingers holding the stick, the cheek or chin should be used as a finger rest.

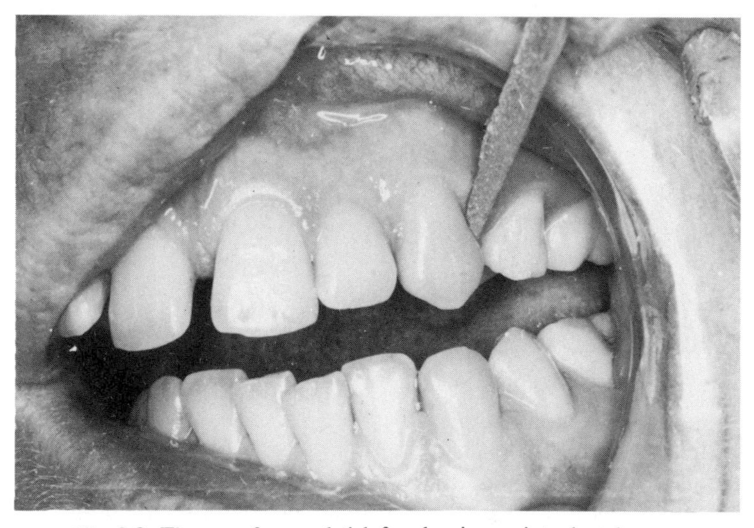

Fig. 9.9. The use of a woodstick for cleaning an interdental area.

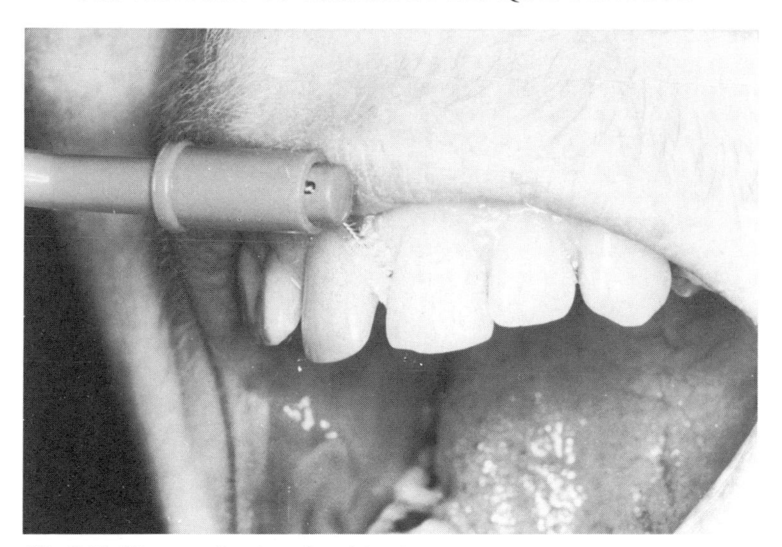

Fig. 9.10. The use of an interdental brush.

Interdental Brushes

When there are wide interdental spaces present, an interdental brush is ideal for the removal of interdental plaque (*see Fig.* 9.10). It is also a useful aid for cleaning around bridges. This brush is shaped like a miniature bottle brush and is available in different sizes (*see Fig.* 9.11). The smaller brushes are usually inserted into handles to make them easier to manipulate. It is important to select the correct size of brush to fit the particular interdental space to be cleaned.

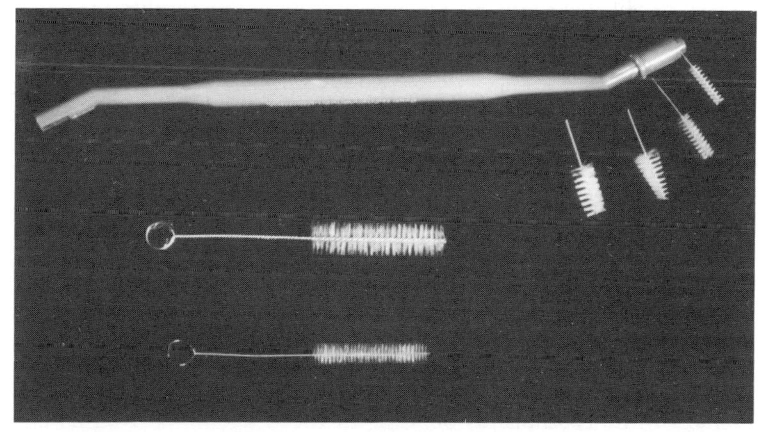

Fig. 9.11. Interdental brushes in various sizes for use with and without a handle.

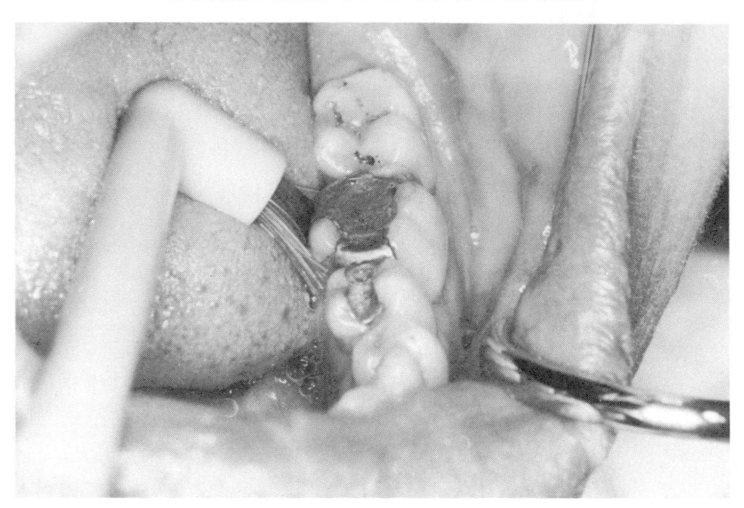

Fig. 9.12. The use of a single-tufted brush for cleaning the lingual surface of a lower molar.

Single-tufted Brushes

It is often difficult to reach the distal and lingual surfaces of posterior teeth or areas where teeth are malaligned. A single-tufted brush (*see Fig.* 9.12) is a very useful additional aid for cleaning these areas.

9.2.5. Dentifrices

In the past dentifrices were used in conjunction with a toothbrush solely for cosmetic and social reasons. However, in the last 30 years preventive agents such as fluorides, antibiotics, ammonium compounds and enzyme inhibitors have been added in attempts to inhibit dental caries. Of all these agents so far only fluoride has stood up to clinical testing for both safety and efficacy. Although the line between the cosmetic and therapeutic actions is not drawn easily, most dentifrices currently on sale have similar objectives. They clean and polish the accessible surfaces of the teeth and provide a pleasant sensation and odour to the oral cavity. They also act as a vehicle for applying fluoride to tooth structure.

Composition of Dentifrices

The basic formulation of most dentifrices is similar. Powder dentifrices contain abrasives, detergents, flavouring and colouring agents and sweeteners while toothpastes contain all these agents as well as binding agents, humectants, preservatives and water. Most toothpastes in the UK and the USA also contain fluoride. A few contain desensitizing agents.

The functions of these constituents of toothpaste are as follows:

a. Cleaning and polishing agents (20–40 per cent). These agents are the major constituents of toothpastes and may consist of one of the following materials:

calcium pyrophosphate
dicalcium phosphate
insoluble sodium metaphosphate
calcium carbonate
hydrated alumina
silicone dioxide
zirconium silicate

There is considerable variation in the inherent abrasivity of toothpastes depending upon which abrasive system is used. However, the hardness of the toothbrush and the force used will also affect the actual abrasion experienced. All dentifrices sold in the UK must not exceed a specified level of abrasivity set by the British Standards Institute. In practice, most dentifrices will remove plaque and pellicle without removing significant amounts of enamel. However, if a hard brush is used with force, particularly on exposed root surfaces, abrasion can cause serious loss of dental tissue.

b. Detergents (1–2 per cent). The purpose of these agents is to lower the surface tension and help loosen plaque and other debris from the tooth surface. They also contribute to the pleasant foaming action of toothpastes.

c. Binding agents (1–5 per cent). Alginates or gums are used to prevent separation of the solid and liquid ingredients during storage.

d. Humectants (10–30 per cent). These agents are used to retain moisture and prevent hardening of the paste on exposure to air. Glycerol, sorbitol and propylene glycol are commonly used.

e. Flavouring and sweetening agents (1–5 per cent). The taste of a toothpaste is one of its most important selling points. In order to mask the less pleasant taste of some of the other ingredients, flavouring agents such as aromatic oils (peppermint, cinnamon, wintergreen) and menthol are added. The glycerol and sorbitol, used as humectants, sweeten the paste. In addition, saccharine may also be used.

f. Preservatives (0·05–0·5 per cent). Alcohols, benzoates, formaldehyde and dichlorinated phenols are added to the toothpaste in order to prevent bacterial growth on the organic binders and humectants.

g. Colouring agents. These are added to make the product look attractive.

h. Fluorides. Most of the toothpastes available in the UK contain fluoride as sodium monofluorophosphate and sodium fluoride, separately or together at a concentration of 1–1·45 mg F/g (*see* Chapter 7.7.1). Toothpastes containing organic amine hydrofluoride are available but have not been tested in the UK or the USA. The caries reducing effect of toothpaste containing fluoride is in the region of 15–30 per cent. Clinical trials of dentifrices containing fluoride in different forms are reviewed elsewhere.[2]

i. Desensitizing agents. Toothpastes formulated specifically to alleviate hypersensitivity around the cervical margins of teeth contain either 10 per cent strontium or potassium chloride or 1·4 per cent formaldehyde.

Mucosal Irritation due to Dentifrices

A very small percentage of individuals are sensitive to some of the ingredients of dentifrices, particularly the aromatic oils and formaldehyde. This can be expressed as desquamation or ulceration of the oral mucosa, gingivitis, angular cheilitis and perioral dermatitis. The practical solution to this problem is for the patient to change to another dentifrice with a different flavour.

9.3. DOES A CLEAN TOOTH DECAY?[1, 3]

A 'clean tooth', i.e. one that is *completely* free of plaque, will not decay. However, very few individuals can ever completely remove plaque themselves, even under supervision. The toothbrush cannot clean occlusal and interproximal surfaces effectively, yet these are the surfaces most susceptible to caries. Several studies have been carried out on the effect of supervised and unsupervised toothbrushing and flossing. The results showed that although there was a reduction in plaque and gingivitis, caries incidence was not significantly affected. On the other hand, when flossing was performed daily during the school year by professional personnel, there was a significant reduction in the incidence of approximal caries.

Dental personnel were also used in another series of studies involving frequent professional cleaning using rotary polishers. The first of these studies was carried out in Sweden by Lindhe et al.[4] over a 3-year period. In this study the children in the experimental group, aged 7–14 years, received meticulous cleaning with a rotating rubber cup and a fluoride containing prophylactic paste once every 2 weeks in the first 2 years, the interval extending to 4–8 weeks in the third year. These children, together with their parents, were also given oral and written information on the aetiology and prevention of caries and periodontal disease and were given oral hygiene instruction, reinforced at each visit. The children in the control group received conventional dental care which included supervised toothbrushing with a 0·2 per cent sodium fluoride solution once a month. The results were dramatic: during the 3-year period the 84 control subjects developed 790 new carious surfaces while the 93 experimental subjects developed only 42 new carious surfaces. The same authors showed equally positive results in an equivalent study on adults. In two other similar studies when the frequency of professional tooth cleaning was reduced to once every 3 weeks and once a month the results, although significant, were not so pronounced.

However, a study in the UK[5] showed no significant difference in the incidence of caries when the effect of professional prophylaxis alone was tested in a group of 11–12-year-old females over a 3-year period. Unlike the Swedish studies, dietary advice was not given and the prophylactic paste did not contain fluoride. Consequently, the effect of the mechanical cleaning alone was tested. The results of another study in Denmark[6] suggest that the frequent use of fluoride may have contributed to the success of the Swedish studies.

The results of all these studies are important in that they suggest that oral hygiene alone, without dietary advice and fluoride, may not be enough to prevent caries. They also show that conventional dental care without dietary advice and patient motivation is ineffective in terms of future caries prevention.

9.3.1. Advice to Patients

What advice should patients be given regarding oral hygiene and caries? They should be told that by cleaning with a fluoridated toothpaste they will, in fact, be applying fluoride topically and consequently be helping the saliva to remineralize early lesions. When root surfaces are exposed, it is important that they are cleaned meticulously with the appropriate additional cleaning aids since these areas are extremely susceptible to decay. However, good oral hygiene, even with a fluoridated paste, but without dietary control, will have little effect on caries. Periodontal health will, of course, benefit if teeth are cleaned effectively.

How frequently should teeth be cleaned? In a *periodontally healthy* mouth, meticulous removal of plaque every second day has been shown to be compatible with the maintenance of gingival health. However, the cariogenicity of plaque is more dependent on external factors: the amount or frequency of sucrose intake, buffer capacity and volume of saliva, etc. Consequently, it is not possible to be dogmatic about the ideal regime for the mechanical removal of plaque that would control both caries and periodontal diseases. Taking all factors into account, it seems that the old rule of brushing twice a day still has merit, together with the recommendation to use additional cleaning aids once a day. In view of current knowledge of plaque pH and caries, it may be advisable to suggest cleaning *before* a meal which may be potentially cariogenic. Brushing at bedtime is also useful since the teeth are particularly vulnerable during sleep, when salivary flow virtually ceases. However, brushing after a pre-bed cariogenic snack cannot be expected to protect the teeth completely.

9.4. CHEMICAL AGENTS FOR PLAQUE CONTROL[7]

Regular daily mechanical removal of plaque by the patient is the established method of plaque control and sufficiently motivated individuals reach a high level of proficiency. However, for many others, effective removal of plaque by mechanical means is a difficult procedure to master. Physically and mentally handicapped individuals may have to rely on others for their oral hygiene. It is also painful to use a toothbrush when acute inflammation is present. Consequently, a great deal of research has been directed towards the use of chemical agents which may inhibit or suppress the deposition of plaque.

If it is believed that all plaque bacteria are potentially cariogenic, then the ideal agent must be capable of complete inhibition of plaque and must be used continuously. However, for proponents of the Specific Plaque Hypothesis (*see* Section 9.1.2) the ideal anti-caries agent needs to eliminate only the specific organisms thought to be implicated and needs to be used only intermittently. Nevertheless, in each case it would have to satisfy the stringent safety requirements for an agent used in the mouth. In particular, it should not induce the emergence of resistant strains of microorganisms nor produce unwelcome side-effects.

Four main groups of chemical agents have been investigated: enzymes, surface active agents, antibiotics and antibacterial agents.

9.4.1. Enzymes

Hydrolytic, proteolytic and glycolytic enzymes have been tested in attempts to break down the plaque matrix and so cause disruption and dispersal of the plaque. So far these attempts have proved ineffective or impractical due to the complex nature of the intermicrobial matrix of dental plaque and the specificity and short duration of action of some of these enzymes. Problems concerning the potential toxicity of some of the preparations tested were also encountered.

9.4.2. Surface Active Agents

Theoretically it is an attractive proposition to alter the tooth surface so that it becomes difficult for plaque to adhere. Studies *in vitro* show that fluoride may be capable of retarding the deposition of pellicle and plaque (*see* Chapter 7.4.2.), although there is little evidence *in vivo* to support this.

Attempts have been made to form moisture repellent coatings on the smooth surfaces of teeth. Silicones and sulphonated polystyrene have been tested with no success. However, with the great strides being made in the field of dental materials we may be able to look forward to a successful plaque repellent coating.

9.4.3. Antibiotics

Penicillin, tetracycline, spiramycin and erythromycin have all been shown to inhibit plaque formation. A study involving children with rheumatic fever, who were taking large doses of penicillin to prevent streptococcal infection, showed a 55 per cent reduction in caries after 2 years. However, such antibiotics are important for the treatment of more serious infections so that the potential dangers associated with sensitization and the development of resistant strains of organisms prohibit their use for routine plaque control. On the other hand, several antibiotics have a limited use in general medicine and are poorly absorbed by the gut. Consequently vancomycin, polymyxin B and kanamycin have been tested for plaque inhibiting properties in the form of topically applied pastes. Of these three agents, kanamycin has shown the most promise.

There is no future for the use of presently available antibiotics in routine plaque control. The dangers associated with sensitization of patients, even with topically applied antibiotics, may be too great for their prolonged use to be contemplated.

9.4.4. Antibacterial Agents

Fluoride

The effect of fluoride on plaque bacteria and bacterial metabolism has been discussed (*see* Chapter 7.4.2). Loesche et al.[1] showed that the use of 10 topical applications of 1·23 per cent acidulated phosphate fluoride over a 10-day period resulted in a 70 per cent reduction in *S. mutans* present in dental plaque. While this demonstrates the antibacterial action of fluoride, the daily home use of fluoride at such a high concentration cannot be generally recommended because of safety considerations (*see* Chapter 7.9.2). Although lower concentrations of fluoride can affect bacterial metabolism, the bactericidal effect of the concentrations used in dentifrices and mouthrinses remains to be confirmed.

Chlorhexidine[8]

MECHANISM OF ACTION AND DELIVERY

Chlorhexidine is the antiseptic which has been tested and used extensively for the control of plaque over the last 15 years. The success of an antiseptic as a plaque inhibitor does not depend only on its bacteriostatic properties. Rinsing or brushing with some antiseptics will reduce the salivary bacterial count considerbly but bacteria rapidly multiply and the count may return to its pre-treatment level in an hour. However, chlorhexidine is one of several cationic antiseptics which, because of their positive charge, adsorb to dental tissues, to the acidic proteins covering the teeth and oral mucosa and to the proteins in saliva. It is the adsorbed antiseptic on the tooth surface which exerts the bacteriostatic action against organisms attempting to colonize. The rate at which the cationic antiseptic is released from the tooth surface will determine how effective it is as an anti-plaque agent.

Besides chlorhexidine, several other cationic antiseptics have been tested as anti-plaque agents. They have been found to be less effective because at a concentration compatible with the oral mucosa they are more quickly released from the tooth surface. Consequently, at the present time, chlorhexidine is the agent which is generally used.

Chlorhexidine belongs to the chemical group of compounds called bis-biguanides which are fungicidal and bactericidal. Its plaque inhibiting properties were first demonstrated by Löe and Schiött.[9] They showed that, in a group of dental students, by *rinsing for 1 minute twice a day with 10ml of a 0·2 per cent solution* of chlorhexidine, plaque deposition and gingivitis could be almost entirely prevented in the absence of oral hygiene. However, in subsequent experiments on unselected subjects, although chlorhexidine was still very effective, its limitations were highlighted. The presence of calculus, overhanging or defective restorations and periodontal pockets greater than 3mm reduced its efficacy since these factors would hamper access of the solution to vulnerable sites.

Since the original studies, using 10ml of a 0·2 per cent solution as a mouthrinse, various vehicles have been used to deliver the chlorhexidine to the tooth surface. The application of a solution at the same concentration but in a *spray* has been tested with encouraging results on a group of handicapped children. Another method of applying chlorhexidine is with an *oral irrigator*. This is a device which provides a steady or pulsating stream of fluid under pressure through a nozzle. The pressure is created by an in-built pump or by attachment to a water tap. When a larger volume can be used, a much lower concentration is needed since it is the total dose delivered and the length of time the teeth are exposed to the solution which have to be considered. When used in an irrigator the lowest concentration and daily dose shown to inhibit plaque formation completely is 400ml of a 0·02 per cent solution. This is a convenient method of maintaining a clean mouth for debilitated patients or for patients with fixed oral splints. Chlorhexidine is also available in the form of a *gel* at a concentration of 1 per cent. This can be used on a toothbrush or in custom-made vinyl applicator trays (*see Fig.* 5.2).

SIDE EFFECTS

a. Staining. The most conspicuous side effect is the development of a yellow/brown stain on the teeth, margins of restorations and on the tongue. The stain is caused by the interaction of chlorhexidine with certain constituents of diet. It is more severe following mouthrinses and in the absence of toothbrushing and is increased by excessive intake of tea, coffee, red wine and port. Professional cleaning is required to remove it but when it accumulates around the margins of defective restorations, it is impossible to remove. This limits the long-term use of chlorhexidine.

b. Taste. Chlorhexidine has a bitter taste and there is a general dulling of taste sensation for a few minutes to several hours after rinsing, depending on the individual. The bitter taste has been masked quite successfully by flavouring agents.

c. Parotid gland swelling. A few cases of unilateral or bilateral swelling of the parotid glands have been reported. However, the swellings subsided when rinsing was discontinued.

d. Desquamation of oral mucosa. There may be individual variation in the tolerance level of the oral mucosa to chlorhexidine. Consequently a few cases of painful desquamatous lesions have been reported. All cases resolved when rinsing was discontinued or when the mouthwash was diluted 1 : 1 with water. Gingival biopsies taken 18 months after daily use by human subjects showed no histological abnormalities.

e. Long-term effects. The effects of 2 years of regular use of chlorhexidine have been studied.[10] There were no untoward lasting consequences. There was a slight change in the balance of oral flora in favour of the organisms that are less sensitive to it but this returned to normal after 3 months.

9.4.5. The Use of Chlorhexidine in the Control of Caries

Much of the original work on chlorhexidine was directed towards the control of plaque microorganisms implicated in gingivitis and periodontal diseases. However, because of its broad spectrum of activity, chlorhexidine is equally effective against *S. mutans*, the prime pathogen in caries. In an experimental caries model[11] using dental students, it was demonstrated that rinsing 9 times daily with a 50 per cent sucrose solution did not result in caries when the students also rinsed twice a day with 10 ml of a 0·2 per cent solution of chlorhexidine. A more recent study[12] showed that it was possible to control caries in a group of children with a high caries incidence and high salivary *S. mutans* levels by the use of a chlorhexidine gel. In this study a 1 per cent chlorhexidine gel in custom-made applicators was used for 5 minutes daily for 14 days every 4 months if the salivary *S. mutans* counts exceeded $2{\cdot}5 \times 10^5$ per ml. A similar regime was also shown to be effective in reducing high *S. mutans* levels in mothers and in interfering in the transmission of these organisms to their infants.[13]

Combinations of chlorhexidine and fluoride have been tested with some success in both children[14] and adults.[15] In the latter study the fluoride and chlorhexidine combinations were very successful in preventing caries in a group of patients who had received radiotherapy in the region of the salivary glands and were consequently highly susceptible to caries. These studies show that fluoride and chlorhexidine are compatible. Since chlorhexidine is more effective at neutral pH and fluoride is favoured by a lower pH, it is not surprising that a combination of these two agents can produce a synergistic effect on caries reduction. Unfortunately, at the moment chlorhexidine/fluoride solutions or gels are not available commercially and since their respective flavouring agents are incompatible they cannot be combined.

Indications

Since there is sufficient evidence to show that chlorhexidine is a very effective plaque inhibitor, should its daily use be advocated for everyone in order to control caries? The long-term unsupervised daily use of any such antimicrobial is contraindicated because of the possible development of resistant strains of microorganisms. In addition the side-effects of chlorhexidine, particularly staining, would preclude its use routinely. Furthermore, plaque is not always cariogenic. Indeed, even though *S. mutans* is the prime pathogen in dental caries, its presence in the mouth is not always indicative of caries susceptibility.

The use of chlorhexidine as an anti-caries agent should be considered only for those individuals who have been assessed to be 'at risk' to active caries (*see* Chapter 4.4). This assessment should be made on the basis of history, clinical and radiographic examination, dietary history, salivary secretion rate and buffer capacity and microbiological examination. In most cases dietary control, good oral hygiene and topically applied fluoride (gel or rinse) are adequate to control caries. However, if these measures have failed or if caries is rampant, chlorhexidine should be used as outlined below.

Patients with greatly reduced salivary flow who are consequently very much 'at risk' to caries benefit from the prophylactic use of chlorhexidine in conjunction with fluoride (*see* Chapter 5.4.2). In the future, if more evidence becomes available, chlorhexidine may also be used prophylactically to prevent the transmission of cariogenic microorganisms from parents to children and from primary teeth to the permanent dentition.

Method of Application

Before application, all open carious lesions should be restored or dressed. A prophylaxis will reduce subsequent staining. Vinyl applicator trays (*see Fig.* 5.2) are made for each patient for the application of a 1 per cent gel for 5 minutes daily for 14 days. About 5–10 drops of the gel are spread evenly in each tray. During application, chewing movements by the patient will ensure that the gel reaches interproximal areas. This form of application is more comfortable and more effective than rinsing with a solution or brushing with a gel since it is not diluted by saliva and is confined to the teeth. Consequently, the tongue and mucous membranes have little contact with it, minimizing mucosal irritation and alteration of taste sensation.

The effects of chlorhexidine used in this way for the control of caries should ideally be monitored by microbiological examination. If it has been successful in reducing the salivary *S. mutans* counts to below $2{\cdot}5 \times 10^5$ counts per ml, the patient should continue to use a daily fluoride mouthrinse to help remineralize any chalky enamel lesions. If the count remains high, the patient has probably not used the gel as directed. In such cases it may be possible to reduce the *S. mutans* counts by applying the gel in the surgery for three 5-minute applications on two consecutive days, allowing the patient to rinse with water between applications.

In some cases recolonization may occur due to remnants of *S. mutans* in cracks in the enamel surface. Consequently, retreatment may be necessary in 3–4 months. In every case dietary advice and oral hygiene instruction must precede treatment with chlorhexidine.

9.5 IMMUNIZATION

Since caries is an infective disease caused by specific pathogens, it can theoretically be prevented by immunization. The association of *S. mutans* with the production of rampant caries in experimental animals and caries in man has led to a great deal of research in the past decade to develop a method of immunization against caries. To date, human studies have not been carried out.

9.5.1. Active Systemic Immunization

Rats, hamsters and monkeys have been used to test the effects of various vaccines on antibody response and/or the development of dental caries. Immunization was carried out using whole cells, cell fractions or cell products of *S. mutans*. They have been administered orally as well as by injection beneath the skin or oral mucous membrane, into the peritoneal cavity and the major salivary glands.

The results of these studies show that immunized animals develop less caries than controls. However, the exact protective mechanism is not fully understood, although it appears to differ in rodents and primates. It is evident that both serum (IgG) and secretory (salivary) (IgA) antibodies to *S. mutans* can be induced. In rodents salivary (IgA) antibodies appear to be effective. In primates, however, there is no evidence that these salivary (IgA) antibodies are protective but clear evidence that serum (IgG) antibodies are effective. The serum antibodies enter the oral cavity via the gingival crevicular fluid to affect the colonization of *S. mutans* in the gingival area.

One of the *S. mutans* antigens most frequently tested has been glucosyltransferase (GTF). GTF is an enzyme which catalyses the formation of sticky extracellular polysaccharides from sucrose. Since these polysaccharides are responsible for the ability of *S. mutans* to stick to the tooth surface, it was thought that antibodies induced to GTF would interfere with the colonization of this microorganism. However, results of immunization with GFT have so far been variable. Although smooth surfaces were protected, it had no effect on fissure caries. Furthermore, this form of immunization was not effective in primates. In these animals, immunization with *S. mutans* cell wall proteins has been more successful.

Immunization with whole bacteria antigens carries with it the risk of inducing autoimmune lesions, either in the heart or in other organs. One solution is to purify the appropriate antigen so that it is free of antigenic determinants cross-reactive with human tissue. A second approach is to stimulate selectively a secretory immune response without stimulating a serum immune response. Rodents have been successfully immunized against caries by oral ingestion of either whole cells or purified GTF, producing IgA antibodies in saliva. However, in primates although a salivary IgA response can be obtained, it is not protective.

9.5.2. Local Passive Immunization

Local passive immunization is an alternative method which is devoid of the possible systemic side-effects associated with active systemic immunization. Its application to dental caries has recently been made possible by the development of 'monoclonal' antibodies to *S. mutans* which can be applied topically on the tooth surface to prevent colonization of its fissures and smooth surfaces with this microorganism.

Monoclonal Antibodies and their Application to the Prevention of Dental Caries

When an antigen is injected into an animal the B-lymphocytes respond by making antibodies to the antigen. However, most antigens are complex molecules which do not lead to the production of a single antibody. Indeed, different parts of the molecule, known as antigenic determinants, stimulate the production of several different antibodies. A breakthrough in immunology was made in 1980 by Milstein[16] who developed a technique for producing 'monoclonal' antibodies (McAb). Such antibodies are specific for a single determinant and are produced by a single B-cell line or 'clone'.

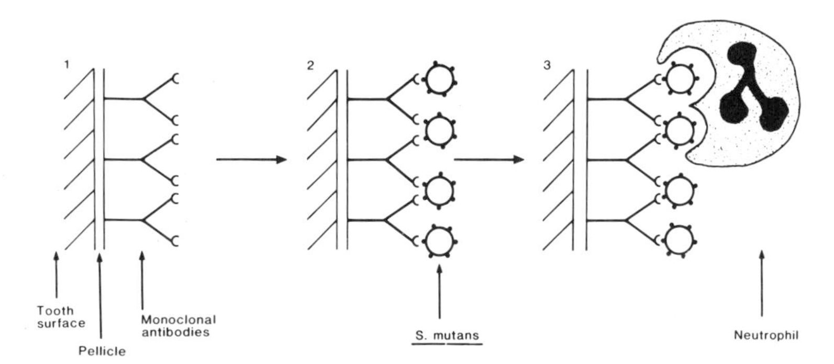

Fig. 9.13. Postulated three-phase mechanism of action of McAb in preventing the adherence of *S. mutans* to the acquired pellicle on the tooth surface.

In 1985 Lehner and co-workers[17] developed and tested the effects of monoclonal antibodies specific for *S. mutans*. Twelve topical applications of the antibodies (anti-SA I/II McAb) to the deciduous teeth of monkeys resulted in decreased colonization of both smooth surfaces and fissures of teeth by *S. mutans* and no dental caries over a period of 1 year. In contrast the control animals showed a high proportion of *S. mutans* on their teeth and developed caries.

Although the exact mechanism of action has not yet been established, it has been postulated that the following sequence of events occurs (*see Fig.* 9.13). The monoclonal antibodies adhere to the acquired pellicle on the tooth surface. Then *S. mutans* binds to the monoclonal antibodies, subsequently enabling the microorganisms to be phagocytosed, killed and removed by the local gingival neutrophils.

With this method of local passive immunization the objections raised against active systemic immunization are overcome, since neither serum nor salivary antibodies are induced. Furthermore, no other side-effects have yet been reported. However, the frequency of application needs further investigation and human clinical trials have not yet been carried out.

9.5.3. Future Research: Questions Still Unanswered

Despite the considerable amount of research being carried out to develop a safe and effective method of immunization for humans, there are many questions still unanswered. These include:

a. Although *S. mutans* is the prime suspect as the cariogenic agent in man, it may not be the only one. Other streptococcal species and species of actinomycetes and lactobacilli have also been shown to cause caries. Consequently immunization against *S. mutans* alone may not confer complete protection.

b. It is not yet known how long immunity will last. In order to be practical active systemic immunization has to last for many years and, like most vaccines, booster immunizations will be necessary.

c. Immunization has to be safe as well as effective. Studies on monkeys provide some of the answers. However, the caries picture in these animals, although close to the human one, is not identical. For example, a great deal more fermentable carbohydrates have to be fed to these animals in order to produce caries. Consequently, we must await human clinical studies to ensure efficacy and safety.

d. If successful, immunization would probably only be used on selected patients who are highly susceptible to caries since the benefits have to be weighed against any possible risks. Indeed, since caries is a non-lethal disease public acceptance of a programme of active systemic immunization may be difficult to obtain. However, local passive immunization may prove to be more acceptable.

REFERENCES

1. Loesche W. J. (1982) *Dental Caries: A Treatable Infection.* Springfield, Ill., Thomas.
2. Murray J. J. and Rugg-Gunn A. (1982) Fluoride toothpastes and dental caries In: *Fluorides in Caries Prevention.* Bristol, Wright, Chapter 17.
3. Andlaw R. J. (1978) Oral hygiene and dental caries—a review. *Int. Dent. J.* **28,** 1–6.
4. Lindhe J., Axelsson P. and Tollskog G. (1975) Effect of proper oral hygiene on gingivitis and dental caries in Swedish schoolchildren. *Community Dent. Oral Epidemiol.* **3,** 150–155.
5. Ashley F. P. and Sainsbury R. H. (1981) The effect of a school-based plaque control programme on caries and gingivitis. *Br. Dent. J.* **150,** 41–45.
6. Poulsen S., Agerback N., Melsen B. et al. (1976) The effect of professional toothcleansing on gingivitis and dental caries in children after 1 year. *Community Dent. Oral Epidemiol.* **4,** 195–199.
7. Parsons J. C. (1974) Chemotherapy of dental plaque—a review. *J. Periodontol.* **45,** 177–186.
8. Löe H. (1973) Symposium on chlorhexidine in the prophylaxis of dental diseases. *J. Periodont. Res.* Suppl. No. 12, **8,** 5–99.
9. Löe H. and Schiött C. R. (1970) The effect of mouthrinses and topical application of chlorhexidine on the development of dental plaque and gingivitis in man. *J. Periodont. Res.* **5,** 79–83.
10. Löe H. (ed.) (1979) Two years oral use of chlorhexidine in man. *J. Periodont. Res.* **11,** 135–175.
11. Löe H., Von der Fehr F. R. and Schiött C. R. (1972) Inhibition of experimental caries by plaque prevention. The effect of chlorhexidine mouth rinses. *Scand. J. Dent. Res.* **80,** 1–9.
12. Zickert I., Emilson C. G. and Krasse B. (1982) Effect of caries preventive measures in children highly infected with the bacterium *Streptococcus mutans. Arch. Oral Biol.* **27,** 861–868.
13. Kohler B., Bratthal D. and Krasse B. (1983) Preventive measures in mothers influence the establishment of the bacterium *Streptococcus mutans* in their infants. *Arch. Oral Biol.* **28,** 225–231.
14. Luoma H., Murtomaa H., Nuuja T. et al. (1978) A simultaneous reduction of caries and gingivitis in a group of schoolchildren receiving chlorhexidine-fluoride applications. Results after 2 years. *Caries Res.* **12,** 290–298.
15. Katz S. (1982) The use of fluoride and chlorhexidine for the prevention of radiation caries. *J. Am. Dent. Assoc.* **104,** 164–170.
16. Milstein C. (1980) Monoclonal antibodies. *Sci. Am.* **243,** 66–74.
17. Lehner T., Caldwell J. and Smith R. (1985) Local passive immunization by monoclonal antibodies against Streptococcal Antigen I/II in the prevention of dental caries. *Infect. Immun.* **50,** 796–799.

CHAPTER 10

THE OPERATIVE MANAGEMENT OF CARIES

10.1. INTRODUCTION

This is not a textbook of operative dentistry. However, a book on caries is incomplete without some consideration of the operative management of the disease. Practising dentists spend a major part of their time, and derive a substantial part of their income, from repairing the ravages of dental caries; holes are cut in teeth and the defects are repaired with all the technical expertise that can be mustered. The dental schools fuel the system by producing efficient cutting automatons, confident of their own technical ability. As the years go by, unless they are myopic or peripatetic, dentists see their own work fail in some patients until eventually the destruction of the dental tissues leads to crowns and ultimately tooth loss.

However, the experienced practitioner knows that when a truly preventive philosophy is combined with good restorative care, the dentition can last a lifetime.

The student's first introduction to cavity preparation is likely to be in the dental school phantom head room. Since the subject is so intimately connected with the study of dental caries, it is to be hoped that the reader is taught cavity preparation on extracted carious teeth, Unfortunately, many students are taught on caries-free natural teeth and therefore come to the clinic well versed in stone masonry but rather ignorant of the disease process. At least they have some concept of the tissues involved, unlike the few unfortunate students who are asked to work on plaster and plastic counterfeits. This chapter seeks to examine cavity preparation in the light of current understanding of the disease process, the dental tissues and the restorative materials available.

10.2. DENTAL CARIES AND CAVITY PREPARATION

10.2.1. Why Restore Teeth At All?

Although the early lesion may be treated by preventive means and hopefully arrested, cavities in the dental tissues will not calcify up from the base. These are plaque traps which are often inaccessible to oral hygiene aids. Consequently the disease is likely to progress unless the sugary substrate is completely eliminated from the diet. As seen in Chapter 6, complete elimination of sugar is impractical. Thus the rationale behind cavity preparation and restoration must be to restore permanently the integrity of the dental tissues, eliminating plaque traps.

Unfortunately, this laudable aim is not attainable because none of the restorative materials available provides a perfect cavity seal and this will be discussed in detail in Chapter 11. This means that if further disease is not prevented, tooth restoration may only be a temporary delay of the inevitable progress of the disease. New lesions may form adjacent to the cavity margin and there may be leakage between the restoration and the cavity wall. Restorations in mouths where caries assault continues are pathways to the pulp.

Restoration of the integrity of the dental tissues is also required where patients are experiencing discomfort in carious teeth on exposure to hot, cold and sweet agents. Caries of enamel and dentine is not painful *per se*, but loss of dental tissue deprives the pulp of insulation and the temperature sensations are partly a function of the thickness of the calcified tissues between the external environment and the pulp. Anyone who doubts this should bite into an ice cream and notice the lower incisors tingle! In addition, exposed dentinal tubules may also be sensitive to temperature and osmotic changes because of fluid movement within them. This sensitivity may gradually subside thanks to two natural defence reactions. One of these is the laying down of reparative dentine and the other is an increased mineralization at the tooth surface due to salivary action. However, in some cases restoration of the tooth is necessary to relieve pain.

Finally, carious cavities are often unsightly, especially in the front of the mouth. Patients, very understandably, are anxious to exchange a brown, discoloured hole for a tooth-coloured filling, indistinguishable from the natural tooth. Indeed, one of the joys of operative dentistry is to be able to improve appearance in this way. However, if dentists do not at the same time stress the necessity of preventive efforts, they are guilty of lulling patients into a false sense of security. Fillings do not prevent caries. They are at best temporary in a diseased mouth and always a poor substitute for unblemished enamel and dentine.

10.2.2. Susceptible Sites

In theory the entire erupted tooth surface is susceptible to dental caries, but in practice the disease tends to present in areas of plaque stagnation, namely pits and fissures, the approximal surface just cervical to the contact point and the cervical margin. These areas are not readily cleansable; the fissure is often inaccessible to the toothbrush filament and to clean interproximally means mastering the difficult, and to some patients tedious, technique of flossing. While it is theoretically possible for all patients to clean the cervical regions of their teeth perfectly, most lack either the dexterity or the motivation to achieve perfection.

G. V. Black, who must be considered the father of modern dentistry, noted the pattern of lesion formation and suggested that cavites should be extended to include susceptible sites. This was known as 'extension for prevention'. Thus, when dealing with occlusal caries, not only was the carious area removed but the entire fissure system was cut out. In approximal cavities the buccal and lingual margins were extended so that the restoration–tooth junction was accessible to cleansing by food shedding. In addition, the gingival margin of the restoration was sited within the gingival crevice since Black postulated, from his examination of extracted teeth, that this was a caries-immune area.

Today, extension of the cavity to include all fissures is not automatic but the decision should be based on the anatomy of the area and the caries prevalence of the patient. Thus the operative approach should be disease-related and tailored to the needs of the individual patient. It is good sense to protect deep fissures in a caries-prone patient, preferably by a fissure sealant, before disease occurs. However, if occlusal caries is already

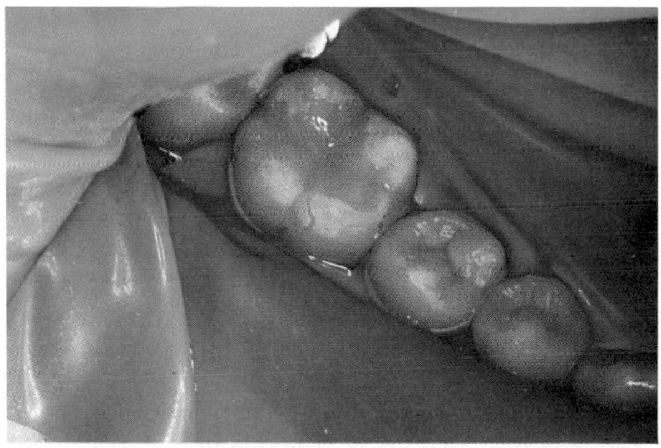

Fig. 10.1. A preventive resin restoration has just been completed on $\overline{6|}$.

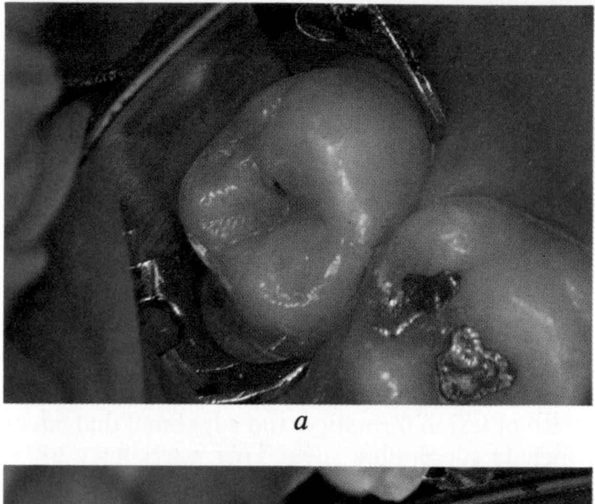

a

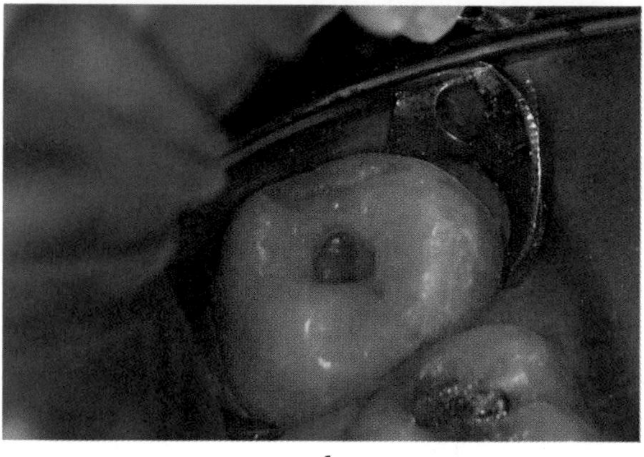

b

Fig. 10.2. Fissure caries which was visible clinically and on a bitewing radiograph. *b.* Removal of enamel to gain access to occlusal caries shown in *a.*

present, not only should the diseased tissue be removed but the remaining fissure system should also be protected. This can be done by extending the amalgam restoration. However, it is now possible to combine fissure sealing of susceptible fissures with filling of such cavities since posterior restorative materials have been developed which are chemically related to the fissure sealants. These materials, known as posterior composites, are tooth coloured and are based on a modified BIS-GMA resin, heavily filled with glass particles to give it strength. The combination of a posterior composite and a fissure sealant is called a preventive resin restoration[1] (*Fig.* 10.1).

Approximal margins are usually sited clear of the contact point because removal of the diseased tissues dictates this. This position confers the additional benefit that the margin is accessible for finishing and checking by the dentist and cleaning by the patient's toothbrush. The cervical margin is not now sited in the gingival crevice for preference since this predisposes to plaque accumulation which may result in both periodontal diseases and recurrent caries.

10.2.3. The Relevance of Pattern of Progress of the Disease to Cavity Preparation[2]

One of the major objectives of cavity preparation is to remove infected and necrotic tissue. Since the disease passes through the enamel and then spreads laterally along the enamel–dentine junction to involve the dentine on a wider front, *access* to carious dentine must be gained by removal of undermined enamel. Smooth surface lesions (approximal and cervical) differ in shape from fissure lesions because of differences in the anatomy at the two sites (*Figs.* 3.1 and 3.2). Thus an apparently small lesion in a fissure is often found to have extensively undermined enamel and involved a surprisingly large zone of dentine.

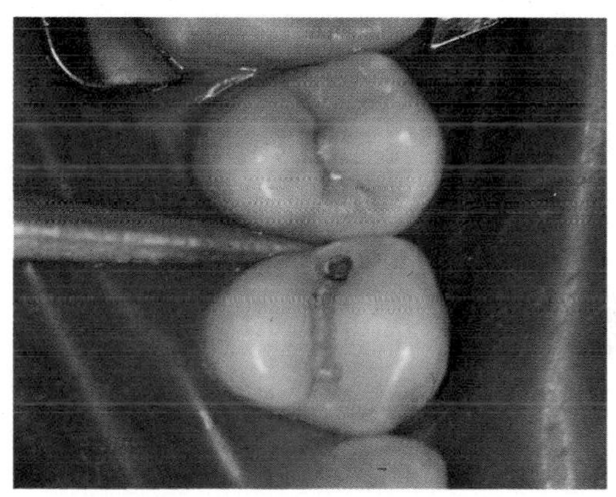

Fig. 10.3. Access to approximal caries (*see Fig.* 1.4) is being gained through the marginal ridge. A small chisel will now be used to fracture away the undermined marginal ridge. This approach makes damage to the adjacent tooth with a bur less likely.

(*Fig.* 10.2*a* and *b* shows the removal of enamel over a fissure lesion to gain access to caries beneath. Access to approximal caries in posterior teeth is generally gained through the marginal ridge (*Fig.* 10.3) which has been undermined by the caries and is destroyed in the cutting process. However, a buccal approach, which preserves the marginal ridge,[3] may occasionally be appropriate, particularly if the tooth is tilted lingually (*Fig.* 10.4), or if the caries is on the root surface and thus well away from the marginal ridge.

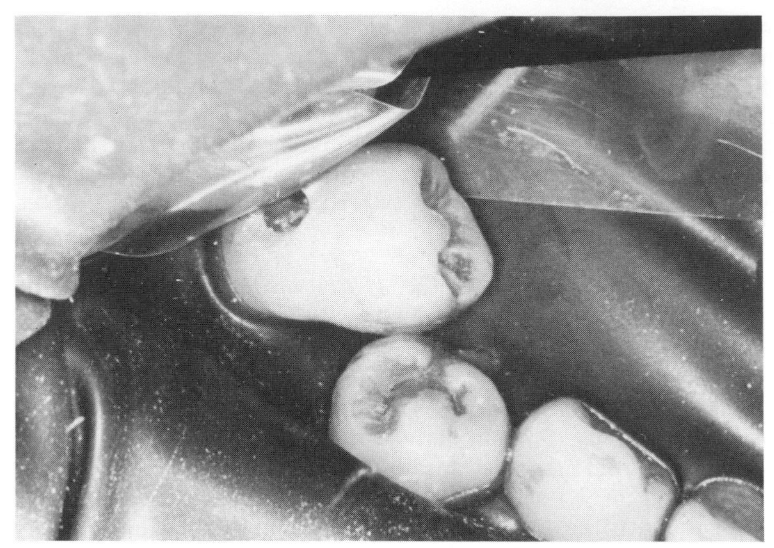

Fig. 10.4. A buccal approach to approximal caries has been used. This preserves the marginal ridge and is appropriate for this tooth because it is tilted lingually. The matrix strip will be used to contour the tooth-coloured restoration.

In addition, consideration is now being given to approaching approximal caries from the occlusal aspect, but leaving the marginal ridge in place (*Fig.* 10.5).[4] This technique is applicable only to a relatively early lesion where the marginal ridge has not been extensively undermined by caries. It could, of course, be argued that such early lesions may often be managed preventively without recourse to the dental drill.

Access to approximal caries in anterior teeth is generally gained lingually so that the restoration will not be too visible (*Fig.* 10.6). However, tooth position, or the position of the lesion, may dictate a buccal approach. Where the adjacent tooth is missing, direct access to caries may be possible.

Having gained access to carious dentine, the *enamel–dentine junction* is made caries-free and undermined enamel removed. It is currently considered unacceptable to leave caries at the enamel–dentine junction because restorative materials which form a perfect cavity seal are not available and the disease may progress more readily if demineralized tissue is left in this area. However, it could be argued that since cavity seal cannot be attained, recurrence is inevitable, even if the enamel–dentine junction is caries-free. The rationale for removing unsupported enamel is that undermined enamel is brittle and prone to fracture under occlusal stress. However, not all cavity margins are subject to occlusal stress (e.g. buccal cavities), so perhaps this is unnecessarily destructive! Despite these

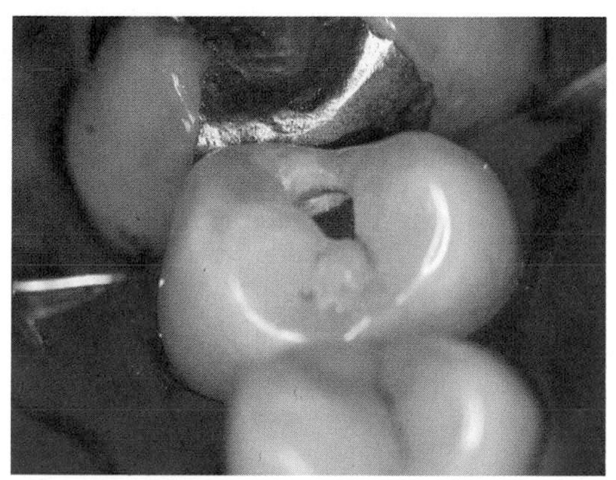

Fig. 10.5. Approximal caries has been approached from the occlusal aspect, leaving the marginal ridge intact.

misgivings, and lack of scientific evidence, it is prudent to remove all caries and stain from the enamel–dentine junction. It may be permissible to leave unsupported enamel in areas remote from occlusal stress.

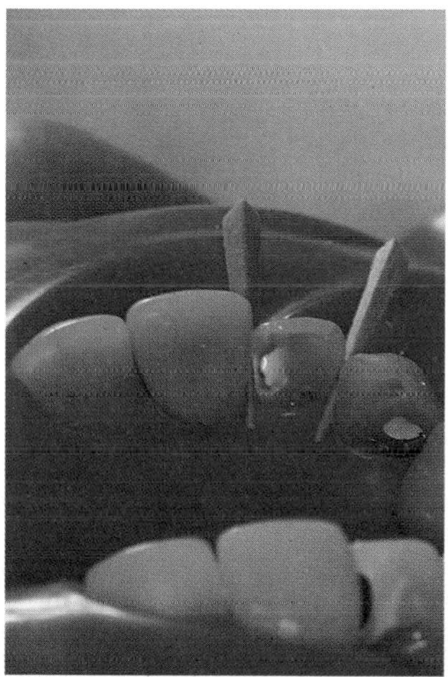

Fig. 10.6. Caries has necessitated the preparation of a large cavity in 2⌋. Note unsupported enamel has been left labially. This enamel will be etched from the inside to facilitate retention of the restoration.

The final stage in caries removal is to deal with the tissue over the *pulp*. Since demineralization is thought to precede bacterial penetration, the interface between the dentine that is demineralized and that which is infected would be an ideal place to terminate tissue removal. This is the rationale behind indirect pulp capping, when stained but firm dentine is left in the base of a cavity in a symptomless vital tooth to avoid exposure. The demineralized dentine which remains is then covered with a therapeutic base material (usually calcium hydroxide) to encourage reparative dentine formation, remineralization of residual dentine and to kill any remaining microorganisms.

The problem of the clinician is to distinguish between the dentine which should be removed and that which may be left. Currently, clinical judgement is used to make this decision, although in recent years a caries detector dye has been developed (1 per cent acid red in propylene glycol) which, on the basis of laboratory experiments, should aid the clinical decision. It is claimed that, with this dye, infected dentine stains red whereas non-infected dentine, which will remineralize under a calcium hydroxide dressing, does not stain.

It is important to isolate a deep cavity from saliva since it has been shown that micro-exposures will often heal by reparative dentine formation provided bacterial contamination is avoided.[5] For this reason it is suggested that a rubber dam be applied routinely when restoring very carious teeth.

During cavity preparation the operator must be aware that reactionary dentine will have formed beneath the caries but will not be present in a part of the cavity that was not carious. Thus, if a cavity is to be extended to include a susceptible fissure, this extension should only be cut to the depth of the enamel–dentine junction. In a cervical lesion the reparative dentine is more apically placed than might be expected. This is because it has formed at the pulpal end of the dentinal tubules which are running apically in this region. It is thus easy to expose in such cavities.

10.2.4. Stabilization of Active Disease with Temporary Dressings

When a patient presents with multiple carious lesions, it is obvious that a combined preventive and operative approach will be required. This approach must include a careful history and examination, diagnosis of the cause of the disease, extraction of teeth which are obviously unsavable, institution of preventive measures and stabilization of large active lesions. All lesions where pulpal involvement looks likely on radiography should be treated in the following way.

The tooth should initially be tested to determine whether the pulp is vital. If it is, a local anaesthetic is given and access gained to the carious dentine. The enamel–dentine junction is made caries-free and caries is excavated over the pulp as described in the previous section. In a vital, symptomless tooth, calcium hydroxide may be used as an indirect pulp capping agent followed by a zinc oxide and eugenol temporary filling.

Where caries has resulted in frank exposure of a vital pulp, removal of the pulp is often advisable to prevent pain. Eventually such teeth require root canal therapy if they are to be saved but initially the pulp cavity may be dressed with a mild antiseptic (e.g. 1 per cent aqueous parachlorophenol) on cotton wool and the tooth restored with a zinc oxide and eugenol temporary filling. Where inadequate anaesthesia or insufficient time preclude complete removal of the coronal and radicular pulp, a vital exposure can be dressed with a corticosteroid-antibiotic preparation before placing a temporary filling. These products are unrivalled in their ability to suppress the inflammatory process and hence the pain of pulpitis, but root canal therapy is the eventual treatment of choice if the tooth is to be saved.

Where grossly carious teeth are found to be non-vital, but the teeth are restorable, the pulp cavity may be dressed with a mild antiseptic on cotton wool and the tooth restored temporarily. If, however, the patient has symptoms of acute apical infection, thorough debridement of the root canal system is required before placement of a mild antiseptic dressing in the coronal pulp chamber and temporary restoration of the tooth.

Stabilization of active, advanced lesions in this way is an essential part of deciding the eventual treatment plan for the patient. It may be that some of these teeth are found to be unrestorable and their extraction will therefore be advised. It is only after such careful investigation that the dentist can estimate the extent of restorative treatment required, such as the number of root fillings. Stabilization also assists disease control by reducing infection and ensuring that toothache is not experienced in one tooth while many restorative hours are devoted to another.

In addition, during these stabilization appointments, dentist and patient will be getting to know one another. Preventive measures can be instituted and the dentist can begin to gauge the patient's attitude towards disease control in his own mouth. If cooperation with dietary and plaque control seems to be forthcoming, a treatment plan that preserves as many teeth as possible will be justified. If, on the other hand, the patient appears disinterested and disinclined to play the essential role in disease control, a treatment involving some extractions and simple restorations may have more chance of success in the long run.

Definitive restorations should not be started in such a patient until prevention has been instituted and grossly carious teeth stabilized.

10.3. MATERIALS AND CAVITY PREPARATION

The materials which must be considered are the remaining tooth tissue (that is the enamel and the dentine–pulp complex) and the materials that are to be used to restore the integrity of the tooth. Tooth and restorative material must be considered together since they abut, support and retain each other.

10.3.1. Remaining Tooth Tissue

The remaining dental tissue must be examined critically to decide whether it will support a restorative material or whether it requires support from that restorative material. Since the forces of occlusion contribute a major part in the stresses that will be placed on the tooth, examination of occlusal relationships will form an important part of this assessment. It is not considered acceptable to leave enamel that is unsupported by dentine in areas subject to occlusal stress. Unsupported enamel is a brittle material and liable to fracture, leaving a gap between the restoration and the cavity wall. However, if occlusal forces are slight or absent, it may be permissible to leave unsupported enamel, particularly if the tooth tissue is itself supported by the restorative material. An example of this is the preservation of labial enamel in a cavity in an anterior tooth that is subsequently filled with an adhesive material (*Fig.* 10.6), such as an acid-etched composite or glass-ionomer cement restoration. This practice has the additional advantages of aiding retention of the restoration by preserving enamel that can be acid-etched and preserving the aesthetic natural labial tissue.

In posterior teeth that are to be restored with metal, current teaching is that all enamel unsupported by dentine should be removed. However, there are occasions when experienced practitioners, having checked the occlusion and found it favourable, deliberately retain unsupported enamel to aid the retention and contouring of the final restoration. It would be interesting to examine, histologically, extracted teeth whose restorations have served for many years. It is likely that such teeth would show numerous areas of unsupported enamel at the histological level. This area of cavity preparation begs for further investigation in both the laboratory and the clinic.

It is not only unsupported enamel that is prone to fracture under occlusal stress. Cusps weakened by the placement of large restorations frequently break off, causing the operators to lament that the weakened tooth was not supported with a cuspal coverage, cast gold restoration. However, the problem is to know which weakened cusps will fracture and which will serve for many years. Apart from knowing that root filled teeth are particularly prone to such fracture and should be afforded occlusal protection, it is difficult to make other rules.

Unfortunately it is not only the carious process that is to blame for cusp fracture. Since the advent of the air rotor it is only too easy to overcut cavities. Dentists are continually replacing restorations; a recent study showed that 50 per cent of amalgam and composite restorations last less than 5 years.[6] In addition, research has shown that cavities may be enlarged by an average 0·6 mm each time a restoration is replaced and thus eventually the dentist simply runs out of tooth.[7]

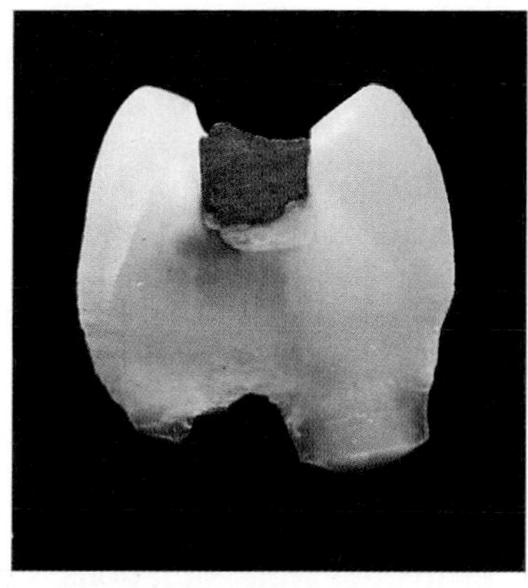

Fig. 10.7. A hemisection through a ditched amalgam restoration. On the left-hand side of the cavity the amalgam probably fractured because the amalgam margin angle was too acute.

10.3.2. Amalgam

Amalgam is retained in a cavity by retentive mechanical features in the preparation such as undercuts and grooves as well as dentine pins.

It is an essentially brittle material which is weak in thin section. It will not support or retain the remaining dental tissues but must be supported and retained by them.

When subject to occlusal stress, sufficient bulk of material must be present to resist fracture. The currently accepted minimal dimensions occlusally are 1 mm in width, 2 mm in depth. The amalgam–margin angle should be in excess of 70°. It is probably the judgement of amalgam–margin angle which is often at fault, producing angles of less than 70° which are prone to fracture leaving ditched margins (*Fig.* 10.7).[8] Ditched margins may be of particular importance because they are plaque traps and dentists have the urge to replace such restorations with a consequent increase in size of the cavity.

10.3.3. Gold

Since a tooth restored with gold is particularly prone to recurrent disease (*see* Chapter 11), a gold restoration, like any cemented restoration, should not be used unless caries has been controlled.

In contrast to amalgam, gold is strong in thin section and is thus the material of choice for the protection of weakened cusps and for veneering tooth tissue (*Fig.* 10.8). To achieve the optimum fit of the restorative material to the dental tissues, a slip joint, such as a bevel or chamfer, is the finishing line of choice with a gold margin angle of 45° or less. This thin edge of gold can be burnished in some alloys to improve marginal adaptation.

Since cast gold restorations are cemented into position, their retention depends partly on the cement lute and partly on the features of the cavity preparation that give a single, long line of insertion to the restoration. Thus, near parallel walls, boxes, grooves and pins are the retentive features of these preparations. Rigidity of the casting is an essential prerequisite for success since any flexing under occlusal load will result in a loss of cement seal and recurrent caries. Sufficient thickness of occlusal gold (1 mm), a chamfered finishing line and internal features such as boxes, grooves and occlusal channels all contribute to rigidity.

10.3.4. Composite Resin

Composite resin is a tooth coloured restorative material, usually used for the restoration of anterior teeth.[9] The material is remarkably strong and can therefore be used in load-bearing situations such as incisal edges and occlusal surfaces. The material appears to have good edge strength.

When the material was first introduced in the early 1960s one of its most exciting properties was its ability to bond mechanically to acid-etched enamel. This, combined with its excellent physical properties, revolutionized the treatment of fractured incisors and the restoration of large anterior cavities where retention had previously been a problem (*Fig.* 10.6).

In addition to aiding retention of the restoration, acid etching also improves the marginal seal of composite restorations. Although it has been suggested that bevelling of enamel margins prior to etching will improve etch pattern and cavity sealing ability, the results of many studies dispute this.

10.3.5. Glass-ionomer Cement

Glass-ionomer cement is also a tooth coloured restorative material and was the first permanent restorative material to adhere to both enamel and dentine by physicochemical bonding.[10] Since a retentive cavity form is not required for this material, it is ideally suited to the restoration of root caries where conventional retention is difficult to obtain.

It has recently been suggested by McLean[3] that this material might be used for the restoration of approximal carious lesions in posterior teeth. Access to caries is obtained either buccally or occlusally, preserving the marginal ridge which is difficult to replace perfectly (*see Figs.* 10.4 and 10.5). A cavity is prepared from such a buccal or occlusal approach, removing sufficient enamel to gain access to make the enamel–dentine junction caries-free. Eventually the cavity is restored by injecting a glass-ionomer type material, using a matrix to mould this to shape.

This is a novel rethink of our currect concepts of cavity preparation based upon the site of carious attack, the problems of replacing the marginal ridge and the new material available. It will, of course, be many years before the profession will know whether such restorations will give long-term clinical

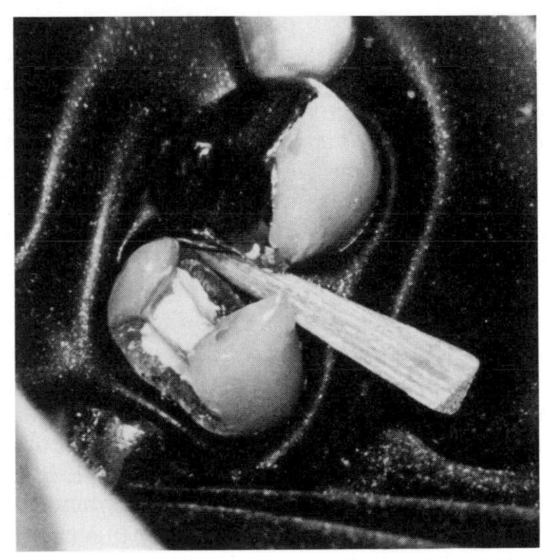

Fig. 10.8. A large restoration has been removed from the premolar. Since the remaining cusps are weak, consideration is now given to protecting them with a gold veneer. The final restoration, after preparation, will be a cuspal coverage, gold inlay.

service, but in an age where fissure sealants may solve the problem of occlusal caries, this suggestion merits serious consideration.

10.4. ROOT CARIES

Root caries presents some specific operative difficulties relating to access and retention of the restoration. Early diagnosis (*see* Chapter 4) is thus of particular clinical importance so that the early lesion may be arrested by preventive measures.

When the lesion is very superficial (*see* Chapter 3), it may be possible to smooth and polish the carious area without needing to place a restoration. On the other hand, if the lesion has penetrated more deeply, operative intervention may be required to remove infected softened dentine which cannot remineralize because the tissue damage has advanced too far. In addition restoration may be required to avoid sensitivity, to protect the pulp and to facilitate meticulous oral hygiene. In anterior teeth restoration of appearance may be important.

Access to buccal lesions may be relatively easy but approximal lesions can present great difficulty. Where root caries is present in the absence of an existing coronal restoration, buccal access is often the most convenient approach. However, where there is root caries at the cervical margin of an existing restoration, access may be gained by removing this filling. Vision is often difficult as the operator is peering down a long dark tunnel. In addition, in the lesion forming cervical to an existing restoration, the margin of the cavity may be well subgingival. In such cases periodontal surgery is required before a definitive restoration can be placed. Access to lingual lesions in the lower arch is also very difficult because the tongue and floor of the mouth are continually in the way. A rubber dam can help, but clamp placement to retract the rubber may be impossible.

Cavity preparation on the root surface may also be complicated by pulp exposure since the pulp chamber and root canal are soon reached. In addition, it is often very difficult to provide mechanical retention for the restoration, particularly in lesions which encompass the circumference of the root. Fortunately, glass-ionomer materials, which will adhere to dentine as well as enamel, are now available. All the glass-ionomer materials contain available fluoride which may have a cariostatic effect. A recent development is the incorporation of silver particles in one of these materials (Ketac Silver, ESPE),[4] making it radiopaque. Scientific assessment of this material is in its infancy but the future of glass-ionomer materials looks bright with new developments continually taking place. It is important to remember, however, that these materials are particularly unforgiving of errors of technique and must be placed in a dry cavity.

10.5. THE FUTURE

This decade is an interesting time to be engaged in dental practice. The prevalence of dental caries is falling in many countries and it is known that established disease can be arrested. However, although it is not yet clear which lesions will remineralize or arrest and which lesions must be repaired by restoration, it is certain that all conventional restorative techniques will fail if further disease cannot be prevented.

New materials and techniques are constantly becoming available for evaluation. It is interesting to ponder what the future holds since today's clinical practice will be merely tomorrow's dental history.

REFERENCES

1. Simonsen R. J. (1985) Conservative cavity preparation design. In: Vanherle and Smith (ed.), *Posterior Composite Resin Dental Restorative Materials*. 3M Co.
2. Jacobsen P. H. and Robinson P. B. (1980) Basic techniques and materials for conservative dentistry: 1. Cavity preparation. *J. Dent.* **8,** 283–291.
3. McLean J. W. (1980) Aesthetics in restorative dentistry: the challenge for the future. *Br. Dent. J.* **149,** 368–373.
4. McLean J. W. (1985) Glass-cermet cements. *Quintessence. Int.* **5,** 333–343.
5. Paterson R. C. and Watts A. (1981) Caries, bacteria, the pulp and plastic restorations. *Br. Dent. J.* **151,** 54–58.

6. Elderton R. J. (1983) Longitudinal study of dental treatment in the general dental service in Scotland. *Br. Dent. J.* **155,** 91–96.
7. Elderton R.J. (1979) A new look at cavity preparation. *Proc. Br. Paedodont. Soc.* **9,** 25–30.
8. Elderton R. J. (1984) Cavo-surface angles, amalgam margin angles and occlusal cavity preparations. *Br. Dent. J.* **156,** 319–324.
9. Barnes I. E. and Kidd E. A. M. (1980) Composite resin restorative materials — a review. Part 2. *Dent. Update* **7,** 273–283.
10. Wilson A. D. (1977) The development of glass ionomer cements. *Dent. Update* **4,** 401–412.

CHAPTER 11

SECONDARY CARIES

11.1. INTRODUCTION

For centuries attempts have been made to replace with restorations the tissues destroyed by dental caries. Unfortunately, the placing of a restoration does not necessarily confer immunity on the tooth and caries may occur in the tooth tissue adjacent to the filling material, causing the restoration to fail. Such caries is called secondary or recurrent caries.[1]

11.2. FAILURE OF RESTORATIONS

Considering the amount of time, effort and money expended on the restoration of teeth, both by the dental profession and the public, it is surprising how relatively few studies have been undertaken to determine the degree of success or failure of these procedures. However, in recent years, research undertaken in Dundee by Elderton[2] for the Scottish Home and Health Department has thrown more light on the outcome of restorative treatment provided under the General Dental Services in Scotland. In many ways the results of this work have disturbed the profession, but present a fascinating challenge for the future.

Elderton's study suggests that half of the routine amalgam and tooth coloured restorations placed in the General Dental Service in Scotland last less than 5 years before they are replaced. These results can be compared with other investigators who have shown the survival time of routine restorations in adults to be only 5–10 years. Thus it is not surprising that 66 per cent of restorations undertaken for adults in the General Dental Service in Scotland have been shown by Elderton to be replacements or extensions of existing restorations. This suggests that millions of pounds may be spent annually on *replacing* restorations in England, Scotland and Wales in the General Dental Service.

Recurrent caries is an important criterion in deciding to replace restorations but it is not the only cause of failure of restorations. Factors such as poor appearance, poor contour, fractured restorations or teeth, also necessitate the replacement of fillings. Unfortunately, secondary caries is difficult to diagnose. In a recent laboratory study[3] dentists assessed the caries status around restorations in extracted teeth before they were sectioned in the laboratory. The teeth judged to show secondary caries in the simulated clinical examination did not always correspond to those which were found to be carious when sectioned.

Since secondary caries is difficult to diagnose, there is an urgent need for improved criteria for assessing restorations. Our treatment philosophy probably needs to change from one of 'if in doubt replace a restoration', to 'if in doubt observe a restoration and reassess it in 6 months'.

Some of the difficulties in the diagnosis of secondary caries may become easier to understand if the histology and aetiology of the early secondary lesion are considered.

11.3. HISTOLOGICAL FEATURES OF SECONDARY CARIES

Histological examination of the early secondary carious lesion gives some indication of how such a lesion is formed. When a filling is placed, the adjacent enamel may be considered in two planes—the surface enamel and the enamel of the cavity wall. For this reason, a secondary carious lesion has been described as occurring in two parts (*see Fig.* 11.1)—an 'outer lesion' formed on the surface of the tooth as a result of primary attack and a cavity 'wall lesion' which will only be seen if there is leakage of bacteria, fluids, molecules or hydrogen ions between the restoration and the cavity wall. This clinically undetectable leakage around restorations is referred to as 'microleakage'.

The early secondary carious lesion in enamel is most clearly seen with the polarizing microscope when ground sections are placed in the liquid quinoline. In this liquid the wall lesion appears as either a translucent zone or a dark zone extending along the cavity wall (*Fig.* 11.2). If the lesion reaches the enamel–dentine junction, it spreads laterally to involve the dentine on a wider front (*Figs.* 11.2 and 11.3*a* and *b*). An outer lesion may also be present (*Fig.* 11.3*a* and *b*) as a result of primary attack on the surface enamel.

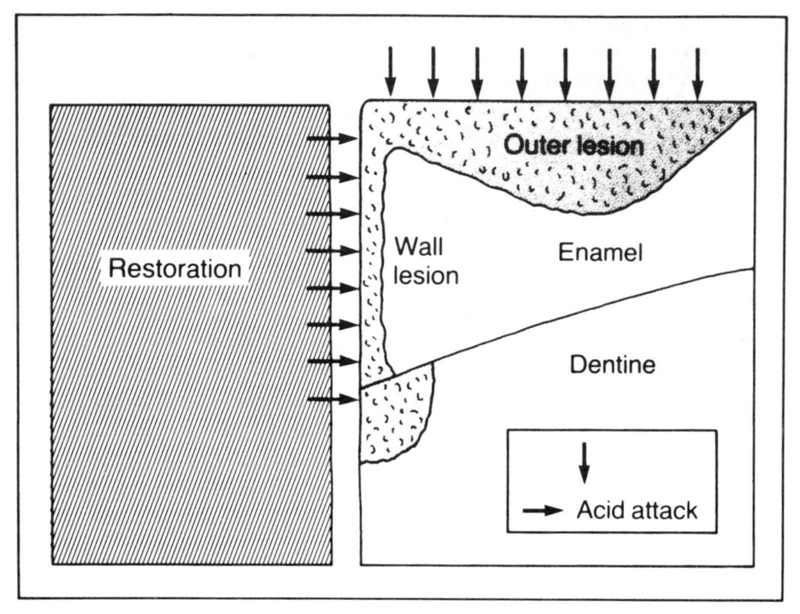

Fig. 11.1. A diagrammatic representation of secondary caries showing that the carious lesion may occur in two parts: an 'outer lesion' formed on the surface of the tooth as a result of primary attack and a 'cavity wall lesion' formed as a result of leakage between the restoration and the cavity wall.

11.3.1. Microleakage

Many techniques have been devised over the last 25 years to test the cavity sealing properties of restorations both in the laboratory and the mouth. These include the use of dyes, radioactive isotopes, air pressure, bacteria, neutron activation analysis, scanning electron microscopy and artificial caries.

Essentially this vast volume of experimental work has shown that all currently available restorative materials leak. This means that if the carious challenge continues, all currently available restorative materials will fail eventually, although some fail more quickly than others! Thus fillings do not prevent new disease and restorative care must be combined with a preventive philosophy.

Studies *in vivo* on premolar teeth due to be extracted for orthodontic reasons have shown that carious lesions can be induced rapidly around amalgam restorations. Class V type cavities were prepared in buccal surfaces and filled with amalgam. Bands were then cemented around the crowns of the teeth to induce plaque accumulation, thus creating a cariogenic environment. Subsequently the teeth were extracted and ground sections prepared for examination. It was found that early wall lesions

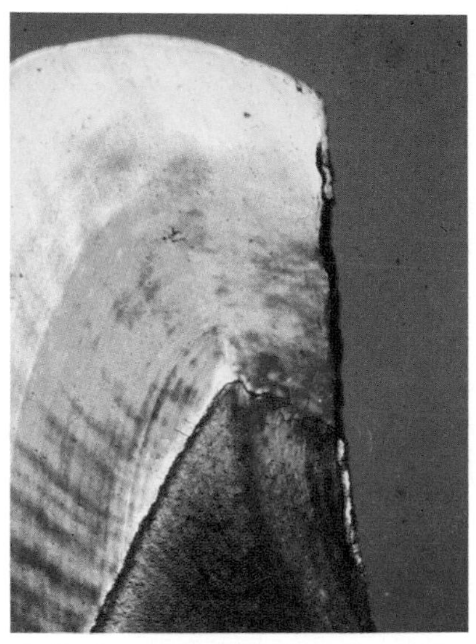

Fig. 11.2. A longitudinal ground section through a tooth with an occlusal amalgam restoration. The restoration has been lost during section preparation. The section is in quinoline and viewed with polarized light. A 'wall lesion' in enamel is seen as a dark zone. Caries has spread laterally along the enamel–dentine juction to involve the dentine on a wider front. (Magnification ×135.)

could be produced around the restorations in only 21 days. This again emphasizes that restorative treatment must go hand in hand with preventive dentistry in order to break the cycle of restoration, recurrent caries and further restoration.

11.4. DIAGNOSIS OF SECONDARY CARIES

In view of the difficulty experienced by dentists in the diagnosis of secondary caries (*see* Section 11.2), the subject is obviously fraught with danger! New caries, adjacent to a restoration (the outer lesion in *Fig.* 11.3*a*), can be seen with sharp eyes provided the teeth are viewed clean and dry. However, at the gingival margin in posterior teeth, bitewing radiographs are required.

The wall lesion, unlike the outer lesion, is not readily seen and is in some ways akin to caries occurring in the depth of a fissure. However, currently we do not know whether *active* caries can progress beneath a clinically intact restoration margin, although on the basis of all the microleakage experiments it would seem likely. Presumably secondary caries may arrest just as the primary disease. Thus the clinical dilemma is not to answer the question, 'Is there caries?', but to answer the question, 'Is there active caries?'

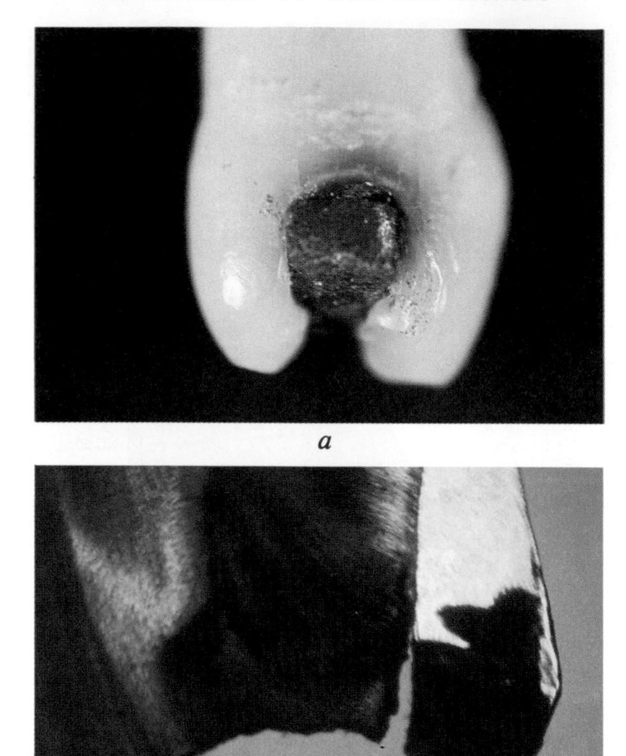

Fig. 11.3. *a.* Secondary caries at the cervical margin of an amalgam restoration. *b.* A longitudinal ground section has been prepared through the tooth seen in *a.* The amalgam was lost during section preparation. The section is in water and viewed with polarized light. An outer lesion is obvious in the enamel. There has been spread of the lesion along the enamel–dentine junction and caries in the dentine is following the direction of the dentinal tubules. (Magnification ×135.)

The diagnosis of recurrent caries is difficult and there are many questions still unanswered. Consequently the rest of this section should be regarded with healthy scepticism and discussed carefully with experienced practitioners and teachers!

11.4.1. Sharp Eyes

What visual signs are there of recurrent caries and how should there cases be managed?

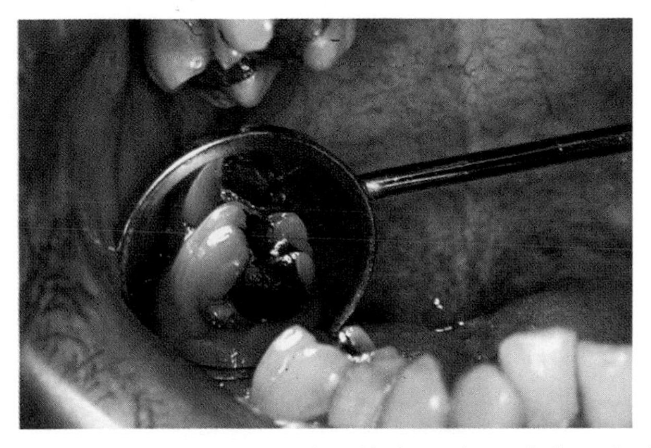

Fig. 11.4. A mirror view of a large cavitated lesion at the cervical margin of the restoration in $\overline{6|}$.

A white or brown spot lesion around a restoration (*Fig.* 2.2) should be noted and managed preventively rather than operatively.

A freshly cavitated enamel lesion adjacent to a restoration (*Fig.* 11.4) should be treated operatively as well as preventively.

A particular problem with amalgam restorations is marginal breakdown or fracture, often called 'ditching'. Although this predisposes to plaque retention and therefore secondary caries, a ditched amalgam (*see Fig.* 11.5) should not automatically be replaced. If there is no evidence of caries the lesion should be observed or consideration given to repairing the defect (*see* Section 11.5.1). When repair is chosen, the whole restoration should only be removed if clinical evidence of caries is found.

Discolouration around a restoration with clinically intact margins is particularly difficult to interpret. With amalgam this colour may be caused by corrosion products and distinguishing this from caries is difficult (*Fig.* 11.6). The judgement is based on the size of the restoration and the size of the discoloured area. A small restoration with a large blue area around it is likely to indicate recurrent caries. A large restoration may discolour the tooth *per se* without caries being present. If, in addition to discolouration, the restoration also shows ditching (*Fig.* 11.7) operative treatment may be required.

All the above decisions will be influenced by the caries status of the patient since recurrent caries is obviously more likely in the caries-prone mouth.

11.4.2. Bitewing Radiographs

Bitewing radiographs are of great importance in the diagnosis of secondary caries. However, unless serial radiographs are available it may not always be possible to distinguish between new decay and decay left when the

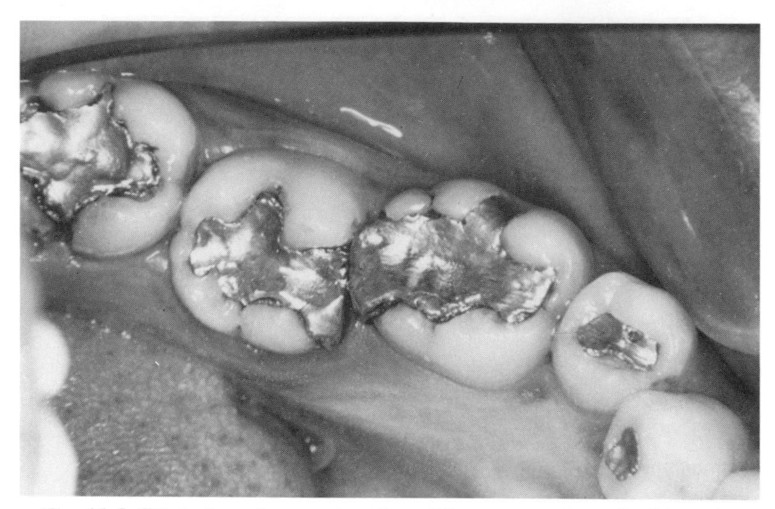

Fig. 11.5. Ditched amalgam restorations. These restorations should not be replaced automatically.

restorations were placed. *Fig.* 11.8 shows caries beneath restorations which should be replaced.

Caries may also be seen on radiographic examination at the cervical margin of restorations (*see Fig.* 11.9). This is usually root caries and may be remarkably difficult to manage operatively (*see* Chapter 10.4).

For caries to be diagnosed on radiographs adjacent to a restoration, the restorative material must be radiopaque. If it is not, the radiolucency of the material cannot be distinguished from the radiolucency of the caries. Metal restorations and lining materials are radiopaque. Glass-ionomer cement is not always radiopaque but the newer cermets, which are glass-ionomer materials containing silver powder, are distinguishable on radiograph. Composites are manufactured in radiopaque and radiolucent form but only radiopaque materials should be chosen for use in posterior teeth.

11.5. THE PREVENTION OF SECONDARY CARIES

It is important to explain to patients that placing a filling does not necessarily confer immunity on the adjacent tooth tissue. Indeed, if the filling leaks, the spread of demineralization along the cavity wall is facilitated. It is thus important that *before* carrying out definitive restorations, further disease should be prevented by dietary advice, plaque control and increasing tooth resistance by means of fluoride. There are, in addition, specific methods of avoiding recurrent caries and these will now be discussed.

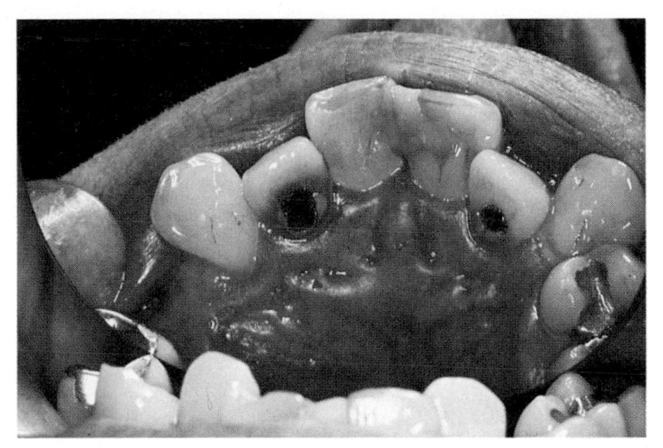

Fig. 11.6. The enamel around the amalgam restorations on the palatal aspect of 2|2 is discoloured. Is this discoloration due to caries or corrosion of the amalgam? A decision was made to replace these restorations and caries was present.

11.5.1. Plaque Control and Restorative Technique

It is well known that caries forms in areas of plaque stagnation. The junction between a restoration and a tooth is a potential plaque trap, thus some aspects of cavity preparation are particularly relevant to the prevention of secondary caries. It is important that the junction between tooth and filling can be cleaned easily. It used to be taught that cavity margins should be finished in 'self-cleansing' areas but it is now known that 'self-cleansing' is an unreliable method of plaque control. Thus, cavity margins should normally allow access for toothbrush filaments, dental floss or interdental wood points. This implies that on occlusal surfaces cavity margins should not be finished in deep fissures where plaque would tend to collect unless these fissures are sealed, as in the preventive resin restoration (*see* Chapter 10).

Approximally, the buccoaxial and linguoaxial margins of the Class II cavity should not be finished at the contact point but brought into the embrasure so that they may be cleaned with a toothbrush. It can, of course, be argued that if patients used dental floss as a routine this would not be necessary. However, finishing these margins in a cleansible area has the added advantages that the dentist has good access when placing the restoration and at subsequent visits he or she can see the margin to check for recurrent caries.

Gingivally, the margins of all restorations should be placed coronal to the gingival margin, wherever possible, because subgingival margins encourage plaque accumulation and therefore recurrent caries and periodontal disease.

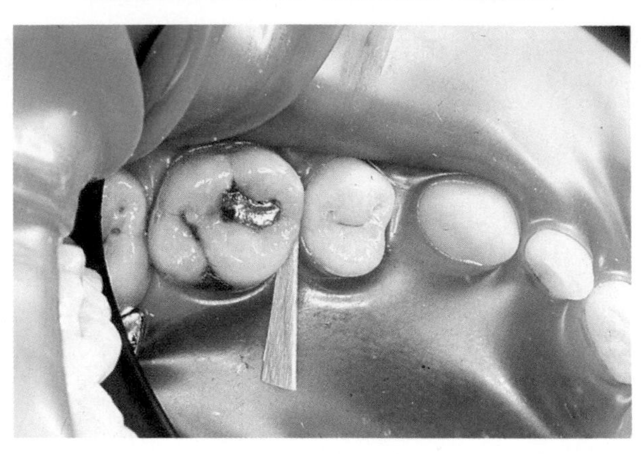

Fig. 11.7. The enamel around the amalgam restoration in this molar was discoloured. The restoration was ditched. Removal of the amalgam revealed recurrent caries.

Ditching is a particular problem with amalgam restorations (*see Fig.* 11.5) which predisposes to plaque retention and therefore to secondary caries. As early as 1895, G. V. Black noted this appearance and attributed it to deformation under the stress of mastication. Recent research has confirmed this observation as it has been shown that those amalgams with the lowest creep rate display the least incidence of marginal breakdown. The new high copper content alloys show a significant reduction in creep rate in comparison with conventional alloys and, in addition, are more resistant to corrosion. Since it has been suggested that the mechanism of marginal fracture is related to corrosion, these newer alloys are likely to show improved marginal adaptation and clinical trials have confirmed this. In addition, ditching may be reduced by attention to detail in cavity preparation. The amalgam–margin angle must exceed 70° (*see* Chapter 10.3.2) as angles less than this are prone to fracture.

Although ditched margins predispose to plaque accumulation and therefore caries, restorations with ditched margins should not automatically be replaced. Research has shown that replacement restorations frequently contain the same in-built errors as their predecessors.[4] Thus, where a margin is severely ditched, it may be more logical to repair that part of the restoration, concentrating efforts on improving it. Alternatively, ditched restorations may be accepted and put under review so that they may serve a little longer. This approach would seem particularly applicable in mouths which are not caries-prone.

Ditching is not the only discrepancy of fit that can hinder plaque control. Overhanging margins, which are particularly likely to occur gingivally, are very difficult to clean, encouraging both caries and periodontal diseases.

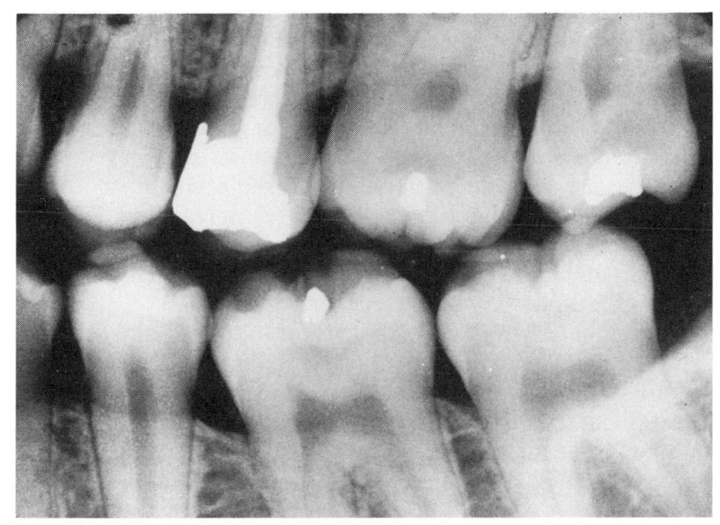

Fig. 11.8. A bitewing radiograph showing caries in dentine beneath the restorations in ⌊6, ⌊7, ⌈6. All these restorations should be replaced.

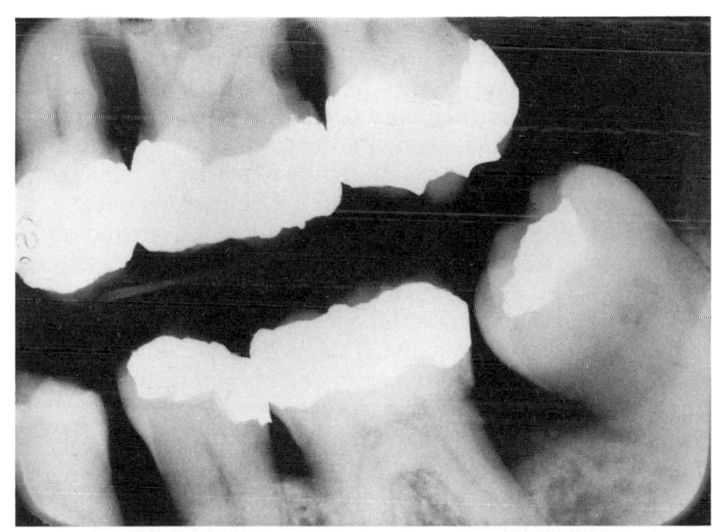

Fig. 11.9. A bitewing radiograph showing root caries cervical to the restorations. In ⌊6 the caries may be secondary to the restoration. In ⌊5 and ⌈6 there appears to be sound enamel between the restoration and the caries. Thus these lesions are primary root caries.

Every effort should be made to achieve a smooth junction between restoration and tooth by careful use of matrix bands and wedges and meticulous carving as soon as the band is removed. Despite all this care, ledges may still occur and be obvious on bitewing radiographs. Such ledges should be removed by grinding with strips or specially designed reciprocating handpieces with diamond coated points or rotary instruments. Alternatively the restoration should be replaced. It is occasionally acceptable to leave a ledge if it is well supragingival, and if the patient is managing to keep the area clean and is not caries-prone. This is a further example of treatment being tailored to the needs of the individual patient; there are no hard and fast rules for every case.

Finally, plaque control is easier if restorations are smooth. Glazed or polished porcelain appears particularly resistant to plaque accumulation. Metal restorations should be polished to aid cleaning. Composite materials are more difficult to finish because the relatively large filler particles cannot be smoothed. The newer, microfine filled materials are better in this respect.

11.5.2. Choice of Restorative Material

Although all materials are prone to secondary caries, some fail more quickly than others. Thus the choice of restorative material may be of relevance in the caries-prone mouth.

Posterior Teeth

Amalgam alloy is the material most commonly used in the restoration of posterior teeth. While the freshly packed amalgam restoration has clearly been shown to leak, many studies have shown that cavity seal improves with time. This phenomenon has been attributed to the formation of corrosion products at the amalgam/dental tissue interface. Thus, the corrosion of the alloy, a property originally deplored by clinicians, may be responsible for its success in long periods of clinical service.

Many studies have shown that the initial leakage around an amalgam restoration may be minimized by applying a thin layer of cavity varnish to the walls and floor of the cavity before packing the amalgam. Little information seems available on the duration of this beneficial effect but it may prevent leakage around the freshly packed filling until corrosion products form and block the microspace between restoration and cavity wall. It would seem wise, therefore, to use a cavity varnish routinely in the caries-prone mouth.

From the point of view of their reduced corrosion resistance, the newer high copper content alloys have posed a clinical dilemma. It is not known whether the reduced corrosion will have an effect on the long-term cavity sealing ability of the restorations. Logically, a cavity varnish should be used with such alloys but it is possible that this layer will eventually dissolve in the oral fluids leaving a channel along which leakage can occur.

Casting gold is an alternative to amalgam for the restoration of posterior teeth. In any cast restoration the gap between restoration and tooth is filled by cement. Thus, the cavity sealing ability of a gold inlay is dependent on the seal of the cement lute. Unfortunately, very little research has been done on the cavity sealing ability of such cemented restorations, either in the laboratory or in the mouth. However, a limited laboratory study comparing zinc phosphate and glass-ionomer cement showed that secondary caries-like lesions were formed adjacent to both materials. In addition, it is known that the commonly used luting agents are to some extent soluble in the oral fluids. Thus, current teaching is that cemented restorations are contra-indicated in the caries-prone mouth.

When the composite resin materials first appeared on the market in the 1960s, it was hoped that their physical properties would make them suitable for use in posterior teeth. However, clinical trials showed that abrasion of the material led to a loss of anatomical form over the years. As far as recurrent caries was concerned, clinical trials carried out in dental hospitals were reassuring but many practitioners reported a high incidence of recurrent caries around these restorations, and largely abandoned their use. It is interesting to speculate why clinical trials and general practitioner experience differed. It is possible that caries-susceptible patients were not used in the clinical trials. In additon, there may have been differences in the way the two groups handled the materials.

With the advent of newer, more highly filled composite materials, designed specifically for use in posterior teeth, the subject has come under discussion again. It appears that the wear resistance of the new materials is greatly improved but resistance to recurrent caries at the cervical margin of the Class II cavity may be poor, despite the fact that they are bonded to enamel via the acid-etch technique and to dentine via bonding resins.

The problem is that these materials shrink as they set[5] and any adhesive material that shrinks in this way will move towards the stronger bond as it polymerizes. Since the bond with the thick enamel of the axial walls is stronger than the bond with the thin enamel or dentine at the cervical margin, a gap is likely to form in this area. The fact that the materials are light-cured actually exacerbates the problem since the surface nearest the light sets first and the material then shrinks towards the light—that is, away from the cervical margin. In addition, the material is difficult to condense accurately within the depth of the box and moisture contamination can readily occur unless a rubber dam is used. For all these reasons, at the moment, these new generation materials should be used with caution for posterior restorations in caries-prone mouths.

Anterior Teeth

When restoring intracoronal cavities in anterior teeth, the clinician may choose to use one of three materials: composite resin, silicate cement or glass-ionomer cement. Silicate and glass-ionomer materials have the advantage of containing available fluoride which will exert a cariostatic effect. For this reason theoretically these materials may be preferable to composite resin in the caries-prone mouth. However, silicate materials are rarely used today because they dissolve when covered with an acid plaque and therefore the newer glass-ionomer cement may prove more durable. This material also has the advantage of being chemically adhesive to enamel and dentine. Where an incisal edge requires replacement glass-ionomer has insufficient strength and a composite material should be chosen.

It cannot be emphasized too strongly that each of these materials is unforgiving of errors in technique. Care must be exercised in moisture control, mixing, insertion, and finishing if the optimum properties of the material are to be achieved.

11.5.3. Patient Education and Review

Clinicians who have not seen some of their work fail over the years are either dental gods or very young. The most beautiful restorative work will fail in the caries-prone mouth if further disease is not prevented. Attempts should be made to find out whether the advice given on diet is being followed and consideration should be given as to whether some form of topical fluoride, such as a mouthrinse, should be continued. Oral hygiene instruction needs reinforcement and this is particularly important where Class II restorations, crowns or bridges are present. Frequent review is advisable in the caries-prone mouth to reinforce prevention and check the integrity of the restorations.

REFERENCES

1. Kidd E. A. M. (1981) Secondary caries. *Dent. Update* **8**, 253–260.
2. Elderton R. J. (1983) Longitudinal study of dental treatment in the General Dental Service in Scotland. *Br. Dent. J.* **155**, 91–96.
3. Merrett M. C. W. and Elderton R. J. (1984) An *in vitro* study of restorative dental treatment decisions and dental caries. *Br. Dent. J.* **157**, 128–133.
4. Elderton R. J. (1977) The quality of amalgam restorations. In: Allred H. (ed.), *Assessment of the Quality of Dental Care.* London, London Hospital Medical College, pp. 45–81.
5. Kidd E. A. M. (1985) Microleakage and shrinkage. In: Vanherle and Smith (ed.), *Posterior Composite Resin Dental Materials.* 3M Co., pp. 263–268.

CHAPTER 12

PATIENT EDUCATION

12.1. A PREVENTABLE DISEASE

Throughout the text it has been stated that dental caries is largely preventable. In addition, it has been stressed that if disease occurs prevention of recurrence should be the principal aim. However, prevention is largely in the hands of patients since many preventive efforts require their active cooperation. For instance, the avoidance of the between-meal sugary snack, the home use of a fluoride vehicle, careful and effective plaque control, all demand a high degree of commitment by patients. For this reason one of the principal duties of the profession is to communicate to patients the knowledge needed to prevent disease in their mouths. In addition, patients may need to be persuaded that their preventive efforts are necessary and important to them.

Thus two facets must be considered in this chapter on patient education. The first is how to communicate knowledge to patients and the second is how to help them to use this knowledge effectively. Communication of knowledge is a relatively straightforward matter, although the techniques still need to be learnt. However, to achieve long-term behaviour change, such as a dietary change, is much more difficult. Should anyone doubt this, consider how many people still smoke cigarettes, despite the well-known link between this habit and lung cancer.

12.2. COMMUNICATING KNOWLEDGE

The ability to teach is not innate, just as the ability to do operative dentistry is not innate. Communication skills must be learnt, practised and perfected just as for operative skills. This section will consider one-to-one communication, discussing *why* it is important, *what* should be taught and *how* and, finally, *when* such instruction should take place.

12.2.1. Why Teach?

Most people are remarkably ignorant about dental disease and this must be an indictment of our role as educators. Since effective prevention depends on patient cooperation the patient must understand his or her role in the management of the disease. This information is an ethical necessity and may be vital to the success of a restorative treatment plan if disease has already damaged the dentition.

It is also worth considering that dental health education may benefit more people than the single patient receiving the advice. Advice to parents on reducing the frequency of their own sugar intake could logically lead to enquiries about a child's diet.

12.2.2. What to Teach

Throughout this text it has been stressed that the management of dental caries must be based on the needs of the individual patient. Health education must be similarly tailored to the needs of the individual, and these needs can only be determined from a careful history and examination. Communication is a two-way process which must start with the dentist listening to the patient.

Careful history taking will reveal what the patient defines as his dental problem, if any. Questions about whether any fillings are present and whether these have needed to be frequently replaced will help to build up a picture of past caries experience. A discussion about diet may reveal a sweet tooth or a preference for sour (acidic) foods.

From a careful history the dentist will gain invaluable information about the patient's attitude to his or her teeth and the possible personal role in the prevention of dental disease. For instance, does this individual see him- or herself as vulnerable to dental disease? How serious does the patient think dental disease is? Attitudes vary over a wide spectrum from little interest in preserving a healthy dentition to an almost fanatical dread of losing teeth. The dentist can also begin to judge the value of teeth in the life of the particular patient. For instance, would this person be prepared to take time off work, and lose income, to attend the dentist? Finally, the dentist may begin to assess the patient's attitude to preventive dentistry. Is this someone who believes he or she can control their dental destiny, or is this an individual who views dental disease as inevitable and beyond control?

Gradually a picture of current attitudes and beliefs will emerge. Then a careful examination will reveal the patient's current dental status. Based on this information a health education strategy relevant to the patient can be formulated.

12.2.3. How to Teach

Do Not Ignore the Obvious

At first sight it may seem unnecessary to advise students how to give health education. Much of the advice is common sense but the role of teacher does not come easily to everyone.

For instance, it is common sense that when two people talk, both should be seated comfortably in chairs beside or opposite each other. The patient should not be lying down in the supine position in which the dentist operates, nor should the dentist sit behind the patient and address remarks to the back of the head. This advice is so obvious it probably seems ridiculous to the reader that it has even been written down. However, the authors are reasonably sure that if the student readers now go into the clinic, they will see some poor unfortunate patient being taught to brush his teeth, or use dental floss, supine!

Understandable Messages

One of the problems in health education is to make the message understandable to the patient. It is all too easy to make mistaken assumptions about the patient's knowledge and the clinician needs to start by finding out what the patient already knows. It is important that patients understand the words used by a health educator. Words such as 'caries', 'plaque', 'bacteria', 'pH fall', 'demineralization', may trip merrily from the tongue to leave the patient bewildered and silent but nodding and smiling to try to show understanding so as not to appear ignorant. When explaining the cause of caries to a patient the explanation must be simple so that it can be understood. At the same time, the educator must not 'talk down to' or belittle the listener. This means that once again the message must be tailored to the needs of the individual. Ways of explaining will vary according to the knowledge and expectations of the listener. Imagine explaining the cause of caries to a chemistry graduate and compare this with explaining the same problem to a child. It is worth spending time considering how the message should be put across to that particular patient.

Amount of Information Given

It is a mistake to try to give too much information at one time since it is then likely that nothing will be remembered. For instance, to try to explain the cause of caries to a patient, to make specific recommendations about their diet, to show them how to use a fluoride mouthrinse and check that they are cleaning their teeth correctly, all at one visit, would be very unwise. Each package of information should be put across at a separate visit.

Thus, the objectives of each education session should be clear in the teacher's mind and the important pieces of information should be stressed and repeated. To give an example, when explaining the relationship between sugar and caries, one of the most important facts is that the frequency of eating sugar should be reduced. The teacher may spend time explaining why this is so but might finish by saying, 'The most important thing for you to remember is only to have sugar at mealtimes'.

Specific and Precise Information

Advice to patients should be specific and precise whenever possible. When giving dietary advice, a knowledge of the patient's eating habits may help to achieve this. On the basis of a diet analysis it may be possible to say, 'What I would really like you to do is give up sugar in tea and coffee'. The clinician can then move on to discuss with the patient why this advice is important and whether the patient thinks he or she might be able to do it (*see Fig.* 6.2).

Written Advice

Written advice can often reinforce a verbal message. A good example of this is in the dietary advice given following diet analysis. It is helpful to write down specific information for the patient (*see* Chapter 6). An example of this might be that the possibility of giving up sugar in tea and coffee has been discussed, and the patient may have agreed to try an artificial sweetener. Names of possible artificial sweeteners should then be written down to help the patient remember what to buy when going to the pharmacist. It is important to record in the patient's notes the advice given so that at the next visit the clinician may enquire whether the patient was able to obtain the sugar substitute and whether it is an acceptable alternative to sugar.

See Them in Action

When trying to teach a technique, such as toothbrushing, it is very important to see the patient in action. No amount of discussion or use of models will substitute for seeing what the patient actually does in the mouth with brush or floss. For one thing, if behaviour is to be modified it is necessary to see how it is currently carried out. There may be a problem of root caries where efficient plaque control is an important part of the preventive strategy. If a disclosing solution is used the patient can be shown the stained plaque at the cervical margin. The patient might then be asked how that area of the mouth is normally cleaned. If cleaning is effective, no more may be said about technique, but if plaque is still present the patient might be shown either how to angle the brush to get access to that particular area or told that the design of the brush may need to be modified. Practical techniques should be taught in a practical way.

Audiovisual Aids

Audiovisual aids are an accepted educational technique. However, the value of a recorded message to deliver a health education message on a one-to-one basis is relatively limited. This is mainly because a recorded message cannot be 'patient specific' unless it is recorded for one person. Not only would this suggestion be impractical but a recording does not allow or encourage the patient to speak and question, and effective communication must be a two-way process.

On the other hand, visual aids can be of great value. The use of disclosing solution is almost mandatory when giving oral hygiene instruction since without it neither the educator not the patient can effectively visualize plaque.

A large mirror is also of great assistance so that a patient can see clearly. Radiographs can also be used to explain the carious process. For instance, if multiple interproximal enamel lesions are to be treated by preventive means, it is helpful to show the lesions to the patient explaining why they are there and how their progress can be arrested.

Evaluating Performance

In any teaching, it is not only what is taught that matters, it is what is understood and remembered that counts. Thus, the teacher must try to establish whether the message has been understood. This can be done by asking the patient to demonstrate what has been shown or to repeat what has been said. However, it is important to remember that questions such as, 'Have you understood?' may not be helpful since the patient is likely to answer 'Yes' so as not to appear foolish. Similarly, questions should be phrased so that the patient does not lose face through failing to learn or remember. The questions should be phrased so that the teacher takes the responsibility for the failure. For instance, supposing a dentist has just explained to a patient how to use a fluoride mouthwash, the dentist might say, 'I'd like you to take the first mouthwash now'. The patient can then be handed the mouthwash bottle and, while the dentist writes up the notes, one eye can be kept on the patient to see that the product is being used correctly. In this way the patient does not lose face and the educator finds out whether the message has been understood.

At a subsequent visit it is essential to check whether a piece of information or advice has been acted upon. For instance, if a patient was advised to try an artificial sweetener to tea and coffee at one visit, at the next appointment the operator should enquire whether the sweetener has been tried and whether the patient finds the taste acceptable. However, achieving long-term behaviour change is infinitely more difficult than the transmission of a message (*see* Section 12.3). After all, patients may understand and remember that an artificial sweetener should be used but may find the taste so revolting that they are not prepared to give up sugar.

12.2.4. When to Teach

It has already been stressed that health education must be problem-based and patient-specific. It follows, therefore, that it must stem from the history and examination. It has also been pointed out that information should be transmitted in small packages.

Where patients require operative treatment, such as stabilization of caries and/or scaling and polishing, health education can usefully precede a treatment session. The few minutes required for a local anaesthetic to work may be sufficient to show a patient how to use a mouthwash provided the patient is not too apprehensive to receive the message.

Dietary analysis and dietary advice, on the other hand, may be more time-consuming and require a specific appointment devoted to discussion with the patient.

It should be obvious that oral hygiene instruction should precede a scale and polish so that disclosing solution can be used to reveal plaque. However, instruction in the use of floss may well be deferred until gross calculus deposits have been removed.

Normally, health education should not be left to the end of a treatment session when patient and operator are tired and it should certainly not be relegated to a shouted comment made to the patient's back on leaving the surgery.

12.3. LONG-TERM BEHAVIOUR CHANGE

It is much more difficult to modify behaviour in the long-term than to communicate knowledge. How can clinicians best encourage patients to accept responsibility for their own mouths? Some of the factors which may assist this process will now be considered.

12.3.1. Personally Relevant Advice

If patients are to change their behaviour, such change must seem personally relevant to them. Thus patients with multiple carious cavities may be prepared to accept dietary advice to avoid further disease, provided they see their dentition as important.

12.3.2. The Attitude of the Dentist

The best advice one can give health educators is to show patients that they genuinely care for their welfare. If care and empathy for another human being are truly present, it will come shining through. The dentist must be seen to believe enthusiastically in the message. Enthusiasm can be infectious!

12.3.3. High Trust – Low Fear

Advice is often more readily accepted when given by someone who is trusted by the patient. Trust is best earned over the years by a continuing care and concern for patients and their families. Thus, although advice may not be accepted immediately, behaviour may be modified gradually over a period of years.

Fear is not regarded as a good motivator; thus to threaten a patient, 'If you don't change your diet you're going to lose your teeth', may not be helpful. A more gentle approach, such as, 'I am worried you may get new decay around these fillings if we don't try to modify your diet', may be more successful. On the other hand, first coronary sufferers often give up smoking and start jogging, so fear may have a role to play!

12.3.4. Praise Rather Than Rebuke

It is human nature to relish praise and dislike rebukes. To praise a patient for doing so well and then suggest how to do even better may be more successful than continually criticizing. Oral hygiene instruction is a good example of this. It is usually possible to find areas where cleaning is perfect. Having pointed these out, the teacher can then move on to give more assistance in areas where plaque is being missed.

12.3.5. Avoid Confrontation

Confrontation is not useful when trying to modify behaviour. Dentist and patient should be seen to be on the same side, waging war on the mutual enemy of dental disease. To give an example, it may not be helpful to say to a patient with multiple carious lesions, 'These holes in your teeth are your own fault; you must be eating too many sweet things'. A better approach would be, 'Let's see if we can find out why you have so many holes in your teeth; if we can find the cause we may be able to prevent more forming'.

12.3.6. Realistic Goals

When attempting to advise on behaviour change, the advice given must be realistic. If it is not, it will be ignored. Dietary advice is an excellent example of this. To ask a patient to give up sugar completely is unrealistic. However, to suggest how sugar may be confined to mealtimes is advice that may well be followed. It is better to set small but manageable goals than to attempt a radical change which may fail. It is also good practice to involve the patient in formulating the advice. For instance, when looking at the diet sheet on page 73, it was the patient who suggested giving up sugar in tea. Dentist and patient then discussed whether this suggestion was viable, exploring possible barriers. This patient remarked that family and friends at work would have to be told about the change so that tea containing sugar would not be given to her.

12.3.7. Scoring

A scoring system that enables both dentist and patient to monitor behaviour change may well be helpful. The use of *S. mutans* and lactobacillus counts is an example of such a system. Once the patient understands the relevance of the tests (*see* Chapter 9) he or she may well show considerable interest in the result.

12.3.8. Feedback

If a dentist asks a patient to modify some health behaviour, an enquiry should be made about this at the next visit. For instance, if the dentist has asked the patient to give up his or her favourite hot, sweet drink before bed, it would be churlish indeed not to mention this at the next appointment. A question such as, 'How are you getting on without your Ovaltine before you go to sleep; can you manage without it?' shows care, concern and an appreciation that the behaviour modification requested is not going to be easy for the patient. If the patient claims to have given up the drink completely, praise is certainly due. However, the patient may say he or she can do without it 'most nights' and here encouragement is obviously called for. If, on the other hand, the reply is, 'No trouble at all, I'm having Horlicks instead', further advice is needed since Horlicks also contains sugar!

12.3.9. Regular Positive Reinforcement

A course of treatment in which dentist and patient have attempted to modify a behaviour, such as dietary or oral hygiene practice, requires regular positive reinforcement. The frequency of such reinforcement should, as with all preventive techniques, be tailored to the needs of the individual. When should this patient be seen again? A week, a month, several months, a year, or more? The decision will be based on the disease with which the patient presents and the response to the dental care provided.

12.3.10. Failure!

A few words on failure seem appropriate since cooperation is not always won. First of all, think positively: there may have been some success! Oral hygiene may not be perfect, but it may be better. Diet may not have changed but the patient may now know what should be done and with more encouragement may gradually adopt new habits. Alternatively, patients may surrender their dentition to the drill and the denture but instill a preventive attitude into their children.

Who is at fault if prevention does not work? It is easy to blame the patient when the fault may lie with the dentist who has failed to communicate. In this situation it is worth trying another person's approach. Dentistry is a team effort and hygienist, dental health educator and dentist are all involved.

Above all, it is an ethical necessity to be honest with patients. If the dentist does not think the patient's preventive efforts are sufficient to preserve a healthy functioning dentition for a lifetime, the dentist must say so. Such honesty may finally turn the tide in favour of health. In the final analysis patients are free to make decisions about their own health and if the dentist can accept the patient's right to determine their own dental destiny, the door is left open for further discussion at a later date.

INDEX